Take a Walk on the W·I·L·D® Side

Take a Walk on the W·I·L·D® Side

Written by

Robyn Harris

Edited by AnnMarie Reynolds

begin a book

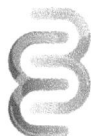

Book Cover by AnnMarie Reynolds (some elements AI generated)

First paperback edition published in the United Kingdom in 2024

ISBN (Print) 978-1-915353-22-1
ISBN (eBook) 978-1-915353-23-8

Published by *begin a book Independent Publishers*

begin a book

www.beginabook.com

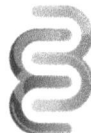

This book is dedicated to:

My Mum - a constant source of inspiration and support.

My wonderfully practical husband, who consistently makes the 'impossible' possible.

All the fabulous animal teachers who have generously shared their wisdom with me on this journey.

And last, but certainly not least, to Geo, who taught me profound lessons about friendship, fun and connection.

Contents

Foreword

by AnnMarie Reynolds

I first met Robyn in early 2021 at one of many 'virtual' networking events we were all still attending. Though we saw each other every week, it was a while before we had a real conversation - during which Robyn told me about the book she was currently writing. Naturally I was curious and when I was privileged to receive a draft copy of the manuscript, I was blown away by its contents. The knowledge and expertise as well as passion that Robyn has for her work is astounding and I guarantee you will not regret picking up this book.

Throughout the many conversations that followed my first read, Robyn and I discovered we had much in common, not least a similar life journey and I remember reflecting at the time on her being one of the nicest and calmest people I had ever met. And that, I think, is what makes her the incredible woman she is today. Anyone meeting her for the first or even hundredth time, would never know how many hurdles she has overcome; she's always the same kind, compassionate, thoughtful and caring person, the one who makes you feel valued and, more importantly, heard.

On the day that Robyn asked for my help in completing her book, I was both humbled and honoured, sentiments that have only increased during our time working together. Many authors find it hard to write about themselves, some prefer humour or fiction over fact and I completely understand why - but not Robyn. She was determined from day one that her story would be part of this book, that she was ready to show the world who she is beyond what most of us see, and let me tell you, it took a lot for her to do it. I've witnessed her struggle as she's doubted herself, her strength and the validity (for readers) of her story. The feelings that have re-surfaced after many years, prompted by her memories have, I know, been challenging. On more than one occasion Robyn has needed to 'take a moment' (she refers to one in this book) but not once has she given up.

The beauty of working with Robyn has been how much trust she has placed in both myself and the process. Even during the walks she has gone on to clear her head, not once has she questioned her faith in this journey and my guidance, and for an editor, book coach and publisher, I literally couldn't ask for anything more.

I am incredibly proud of the work Robyn has done to bring this book to all of you, and I will forever be grateful to her for allowing me to be a small part of this journey. Please, read, enjoy and embrace W·I·L·D®.

Acknowledgements

To everyone who has supported me so patiently throughout this journey—asking about the book, encouraging me, and maintaining a strong belief in my ability to produce something of value—I am deeply grateful. Your steadfast support has been a pillar of strength and motivation. Thank you for believing in me and the message of this book.

Infinite gratitude to Mother Nature—direct, power-full, and fierce at times, yet always loving, compassionate, and gentle. She is my patient and wise Teacher, Guide, Confidant, and Cheerleader. Without her, W·I·L·D® would never have blossomed into existence.

Special thanks to my wonderful editor, AnnMarie Reynolds of beginabook.com. Her invaluable help, support, and encouragement, along with her willingness to challenge me, have been instrumental in shaping this book into one that's not only easy to read and follow but also rich with practical, effective exercises.

AnnMarie,
Your dedication and expertise have truly made
this journey a joy. Thank you for being such an
integral part of bringing this vision to life.

A Welcome Note from Robyn

Hello, and welcome to the vibrant world of "Take a Walk on the W·I·L·D® Side"!

I'm thrilled you've chosen to embark on this wellbeing journey with me. As a token of my appreciation, I've got a little something special for you – a personal pledge bookmark and a nifty screensaver.

♡Bookmark♡

Print it out, complete the easy-to-follow instructions and tuck the bookmark into the book. Let it be a daily reminder of your commitment to your wellbeing.
Feel free to scribble notes, highlight, and make the book uniquely yours.

♡Screensaver♡

Download and set it as a daily backdrop on your digital devices. Let it be a visual cue, a moment of reflection amidst the hustle and bustle of life.

You can grab your freebies right here:
- bookmark – https://equenergy.com/bookmark
- screensaver:
  - ◊ laptop / PC – https://equenergy.com/screensaver1
  - ◊ mobile phone – https://equenergy.com/screensaver2

Remember, this journey is yours, and these little companions are here to support you along the way. Feel free to share them with fellow explorers – the more, the merrier!

Sending you waves of positive energy and a sprinkle of W·I·L·D® magic as you start this exciting adventure.

Warmly,

Robyn ♥

Glossary

Throughout this book, I use terminology specific to my training and understanding. Some of these terms may be unfamiliar, so I have added some basic information on any that I feel it would be beneficial to define.

Life Force ~ the energetic force within each one of us that inspires us to experience, learn, grow, and evolve. It is our motivation, our purpose, and our zest for life and is intimately connected to our sense of wellbeing.

Absolute Self ~ as human beings, we exist in a relative world full of contrasts (light and dark, hot and cold, etc); however, there is also a part of us which is 'outside' of this – which just 'is' without any contrast or 'other'. Tuning into this perspective can help us to explore the big existential questions (such as, why am I here? What is Life all about?) and also our sense of perspective and priorities.

Getting curious ~ means consciously observing, noticing, and exploring everything in our lives with childlike eyes of wonder and curiosity and putting aside any sense of judgment, criticism, or cynicism.

Balance-ing ~ an ongoing, dynamic practice of recovering, reviewing, maintaining and supporting our sense of inner equilibrium.

Dis-ease ~ not merely illness but any form of discomfort or 'lack of ease' we might be experiencing.

Self-talk ~ our inner language. It can be both verbal (thoughts) and kinaesthetic (our posture and body language).

Take a Walk on the W·I·L·D® Side

When preparing for a journey, we often spend time thinking about what we might need to bring with us. In a sense, this journey is no different and, like many trips, the aim is to travel light because W·I·L·D® is all about creating a sense of lightness as we walk along Life's path, by which I mean:

- not taking things too seriously
- being gentle with ourselves
- and doing our best to bring fun and joy into every day - and even into each activity

i. Before you start

As you embark on this adventure, I encourage you to see it as a gift you give yourself – a time for You to be with Yourself in a supportive and loving way. As part of this, I invite you to begin by obtaining a beautiful notebook[1] or file in which to make notes, work through the exercises and record your thoughts and questions as they arise. You might also like to journal as part of this process of exploration into your Self. I know I personally have found journaling both supportive and enlightening.

You might be someone who likes to read a book from cover to cover - this is how the book was written, and my editor, AnnMarie, and I have worked diligently to ensure each chapter flows from one to the next to offer a smooth and seamless path to follow. Reading it this way will

---

1   This is an investment in yourself so choose a book or file which reflects this and that reminds you, each time you use it, of your worth and your reasons for taking this journey.

help you to lay a strong foundation on which to build your wellbeing practice – this book will support you as a guide - or you might wish to jump straight to the core of the book and explore the concept of W·I·L·D® with all it has to share.

Whichever route you choose, it's all good. This journey is yours and you get to decide the itinerary and the pace. Just remember, there is no rush; it's not a competition; there are no expectations, no tests and no assessments. This is an adventure in which you cannot fail. Each apparent detour is just an opportunity for learning and growth.

First step:

Before reading this book, I recommend journaling on the following:

- Describe your current situation exploring:
    * what's going well/supporting you?
    * what's not going so well - things you'd like to change.

- What would you like to achieve along your wellbeing journey?

- What are your reasons for seeking to make these changes at this time?

The answers to these questions will:

- Help you to identify supportive factors and resources you can draw on.
- Give you a benchmark to refer back to so you can see how far you've come.
- Clarify your goals.
- Gently remind you of your motivation should you ever feel you've run out of energy and don't have the strength to carry on.

ii. Navigation

To help you navigate the book, each chapter begins with a brief guide to what you'll find within that section and finishes with a short summary to remind you of the points covered. You might like to start by reading these summaries to map out your personal wellbeing path.

You'll also notice that I've used some symbols to assist you in picking out certain key aspects of the text:

◆ **Exercises**

☆ **Tips** and **Insights**

Below you'll also find a list of the exercises and diagrams as a quick reference:

iii. Some Points To Remember As You Begin Your Journey

- As I said at the beginning, when preparing for a journey, we often spend time thinking about what we might need to bring with us. In a sense, this journey is no different and, like many trips, the aim is to travel light because W·I·L·D® is all about creating a sense of lightness as we walk along Life's path, by which I mean:

    *   not taking things too seriously
    *   being gentle with ourselves
    *   and doing our best to bring fun and joy into every day – and even into each activity

- This is a practice, and as such, it's a continual work in progress. We're human beings living in a fast-paced and demanding world. We get tired, distracted and off balance at times. We're not always at our best. We make mistakes. But W·I·L·D® is about learning to forgive ourselves, to show ourselves compassion as we gently get curious and explore our reactions and behaviours to see what wisdom they might have to share. This is between You and You. It's your personal exploration. You can share it with others if you choose or keep it as an internal dialogue – it's entirely up to you.

- The more you put into this process, the more you will get out of it. I'm not referring to effort as such, but more to commitment[1], time, and embodiment of the tools and practices you choose to engage with. It's more about the be-ing rather than the do-ing, and about exploring and practising rather than being perfect - but this still requires a degree of consistency and focus. There will be times when it feels like a struggle – when you feel like you're getting nowhere and there is no light at the end of the tunnel. This is all part of the process. At times like this it's enough to remember just to breathe! Take the pressure off. Be gentle with yourself. Hang in there and know that this will pass. Tomorrow is a new day and a fresh start. And often, the darkest hour is the one just before dawn breaks through.

---

1 *See the free downloadable gift in the Note from Robyn on pg*

- We are all unique individuals, and each person's experience is different. People may be coming to this book at varying points in their journey.

So, whether:

* you're just starting out and exploring some of the concepts for the first time
* you've been travelling for a while and feel you've lost your way
* or your energy or morale is flagging, and you're looking for a bit of a boost to find your next steps

I hope you find the encouragement, inspiration and support you're looking for.

A book, once printed, is a static thing. It is, necessarily, written for a generalised audience, and while I hope each reader can identify with what I share and find some answers to their questions and guidance for their journey, it will not be the bespoke message to address their specific situation or health issue. I, therefore, encourage you to be conscious of your own wellbeing as you read this book and to do what you need to do to take good care of Yourself. If at any point you start to feel overwhelmed, press Pause, take a break, practice some self-care and perhaps reach out for some support, either from a trusted friend or from a professional.

(I'll be looking at self-care in more detail as we dive into this journey but a good first step would be to read the section on *Safety* in Chapter 3 – see page 87.)

iv. Starting Your Own Journey - The 'Quick Start' Flowchart

Before we delve into the depths of the book, I'd like to share an overview of the W·I·L·D® approach. I want you to see how beneficial this system really is by sharing a simple flowchart that gives you a feel for what your journey may involve and what you can expect to gain. I'm also going to share a personal example of how I myself used W·I·L·D® only recently when I came across an uncomfortable challenge during the writing of this book.

The flowchart uses tools that I have found key during my work and personal growth. These all form part of a firm foundation that will help each of you move forward. We need that foundation to build towards and ultimately arrive at the experience of deep and lasting healing.

Remember, though, at the start of any journey of discovery, we are all beginners, and as such, it's okay to make mistakes. When we give ourselves permission not to be 'perfect', the whole learning process becomes so much easier to navigate because we are not setting ourselves up for failure. We are already acknowledging that we won't always get it right.

With everything I have learned, I believe that it's not about what we do in our lives but about how we do it. And now, it's time for you to start your own journey.

> **TIP:** Before going any further, it's good to make sure you're clear on your own personal values. If you haven't already done so, I would suggest working through the exercise on page 137 first.

Taking that first step

I want you to think of this book as your constant companion, keeping you safe and holding you close as you take those difficult first steps. They may be small, they may feel insignificant, and they will almost certainly feel scary, but by embracing W·I·L·D® and allowing yourself to trust, you will slowly and steadily move away from the negative bias with which we are all wired, and instead, focus your attention on the things that are uplifting and bring you joy. And who doesn't want to achieve that?

So, let's begin!

The Flowchart

The first question asked is if we are experiencing the wellbeing we desire. Before answering that, I think it would be beneficial first to decide what wellbeing means to you. This will ensure that your onward journey has a focus and destination.

Think:

- What does it mean for your body to feel 'well'?
- How would your body feel?
- What thoughts might you have about your life? Or about yourself?
- How would you spend your time?
- What difference would this make for you?

At this point, I want you to ignore any negative inner talk. We will cover our inner dialogue and its effect in much more detail later, but for now, try to answer these questions based on your gut feeling, regardless of what 'other influences' might wish to add.

Once you've made a note of what wellbeing means to you – you're ready to start the flowchart.

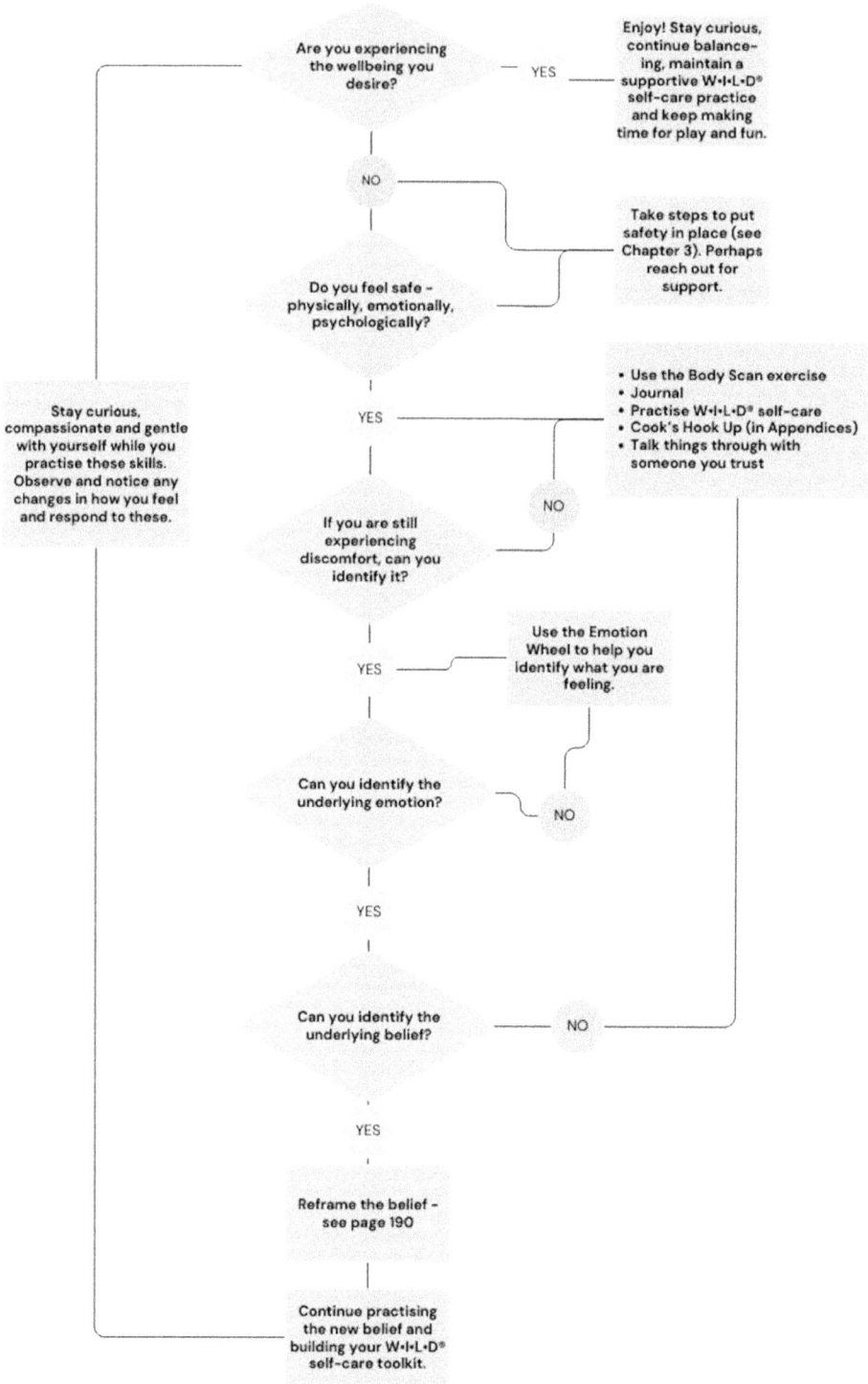

Are you experiencing the wellbeing you desire?

— YES → Enjoy! Stay curious, continue balancing, maintain a supportive W•I•L•D® self-care practice and keep making time for play and fun.

NO

Do you feel safe – physically, emotionally, psychologically?

→ Take steps to put safety in place (see Chapter 3). Perhaps reach out for support.

YES

If you are still experiencing discomfort, can you identify it?

NO → • Use the Body Scan exercise
• Journal
• Practise W•I•L•D® self-care
• Cook's Hook Up (in Appendices)
• Talk things through with someone you trust

Stay curious, compassionate and gentle with yourself while you practise these skills. Observe and notice any changes in how you feel and respond to these.

YES

Can you identify the underlying emotion?

NO → Use the Emotion Wheel to help you identify what you are feeling.

YES

Can you identify the underlying belief?

NO

YES

Reframe the belief – see page 190

Continue practising the new belief and building your W•I•L•D® self-care toolkit.

Understanding the Flowchart and W·I·L·D® Process

Q1: Are you experiencing the wellbeing you desire?

> If your answer is '**Yes**', this is wonderful, and you can give yourself permission to fully experience this and enjoy it – but stay observant because life is full of change and can often throw unexpected curve balls.

> If your answer is '**No**', this is also wonderful because you are in absolutely the right place to make a positive change. This is what W·I·L·D® is all about. Move confidently onto the next stage.

Q2: Do you feel safe – physically, emotionally, psychologically?

> This is trickier to answer but try thinking about how safe you feel in your environment and what kind of emotional support network you have in place. Do you have the ability to achieve inner healing right now?

> If you answered '**Yes**', that's great. It means you have a good foundation in place to begin the work, so now it's time to move on to the discomforts you are feeling.

> If you answered '**No**', then I encourage you to read Chapter 3 at this point. Chapter 3 covers safety in detail and provides crucial guidance and advice, especially in relation to the importance of safety and how you can achieve it. Once you have a level of safety, you can return to the flowchart at any time.

Q3: Are you still experiencing discomfort? Can you identify it?

> If you answer '**Yes**' here, you can move on to the next stage, which will help you to dig deeper into the origins of this discomfort.

> If you answered '**No**', then it's time to use some tools to explore what is going on. Sometimes, we just have the feeling that things are 'off', but we don't know why, so try using things like the Body

Scan exercise I have suggested to get more of a feel for what your discomfort might be. Then, you can return to the flowchart at any time.

Q4: *Can you identify the underlying emotion?*

If you answered '**Yes**', you can follow the chart to the next stage and discover what ideas you may have formed around this emotion.

If you answered '**No**,' that's completely understandable. It can be difficult to determine what exactly feels off balance and the emotions which come up in relation to it. Thinking about, describing, acknowledging, and talking about your emotions can be one of the most difficult parts of this process, so I would definitely encourage you to use the Emotion Wheel (in Appendix 6). You can then return to the flowchart at any time.

Q5: *Can you identify the underlying belief?*

If you are able to answer '**Yes**' here, that's fantastic. It means that you are already in tune with your body, thoughts and emotions; now, you just need to re-frame these beliefs to achieve the positive outcome you desire. From here, you can simply navigate to page 190, where I explain how to do this.

If your answer is '**No**' to this question, it's a good idea to return to some of the exploratory exercises. Working out your main values can be really helpful here because they play such a huge part in creating your beliefs. This may lead to a realisation of values that are in direct conflict with one another, which in turn can lead to discomfort and cognitive dissonance. If you can identify this /these belief(s), you can consider if it/they have a positive or negative impact – does it feel a burden to you, for example? If so, we can turn to tools such as those helping you to reframe your beliefs (page 190), or you can introduce a self-care routine that will turn those negatives upside down. You can then return to the flowchart if and when you need to.

Q6: Continue practicing the new belief and building your W·I·L·D® self-care toolkit

> Congratulations! You've completed the flowchart and are well your way to achieving the state of wellbeing you identified at the beginning.

From here, it's a matter of incorporating this into your daily practice, on perhaps by creating affirmations (which I often call 'Power Truths'), using techniques such as mindfulness or EFT, or following the exercises I share later in this book.

The steps of the flowchart might seem simple, but they are not always easy. I believe it's important to break everything down into manageable steps – you don't need to complete the flowchart in one session or even one day. It's there as a constant guide to help you keep moving forward and to illustrate how the W·I·L·D® concept works.

All I ask is that you make a daily commitment to yourself and take small steps to address whatever you find along the way.

How I used W·I·L·D® very recently!

I promised to share an example of what this process might look like in practice, so I have chosen to use a real-life, personal example taken from my experience when writing this book. Turn the page to read all about it!

My wonderful editor, AnnMarie, has been a great support throughout this whole process, sharing suggestions of how I can make the book the best it can be, however, I was feeling completely stuck on one aspect of her most recent request. To my mind, I had already addressed the issue, and when AnnMarie brought it up again, I was taken right back to when I was at school, and a piece of homework would be returned covered in red pen with instructions to 'Do it again!' But I felt I had already done my best and given my utmost, and it seemed I was being told that this still wasn't good enough!

I have to confess I had a bit of a meltdown. Then I remembered I now have the tools to explore this, so having given my inner child some space to throw her tantrum (which I now understand translates as 'express her fears and upset'), I took action.

I could immediately answer the first question in the flowchart – No, I very definitely was not experiencing the wellbeing I desired! I also recognised that when I was feeling triggered and taken back to the memory of school, I did not feel safe. So, my action started there.

I went for a walk with the dog, and as I walked, I started tapping (using the EFT – Emotional Freedom Technique – we will explore this a bit later) to dial down the maelstrom of feelings within me. This activity helped me feel more in control and restored sufficient clarity for me to identify my discomfort and the emotions and beliefs underlying it.

As I completed my walk, I realised that I was experiencing the fear of failure which brought up another fear – that of rejection and shame. I found this deeply painful because it took me right back to my childhood belief of 'I'm not good enough, so no one loves me' (you'll learn my story in the next few chapters).

Having identified the underlying belief, I was then able to address it. Thankfully, this is one I have already worked on, so I reframed it and dug into my stock of evidence that supports the fact (not the belief) that I am deeply loved and supported by people I love and respect in return.

I now took this a stage further and reminded myself that I believe, with the very core of my being, I am who I'm meant to be. I have a place in this world, and the Universe is supporting me every step of the way.

Reaching this depth of belief has taken time, and, as you can see from the example above, I'm still a work in progress, but that's okay. I believe that's what this life is all about – experiencing, exploring and growing. It's not uncommon to find ourselves facing issues that feel very familiar and, many times, we may think that we've already dealt with them and if we appear to be experiencing the same issue again we can be left with the impression that we 'failed' first time around.

However, I believe we've uncovered a deeper layer. Perhaps initially, we fixed a surface layer or two, but we were not yet ready for the next step. The fact that the issue has arisen again means we've grown, and we now have the tools for this deeper layer - which, to me, is something to celebrate. We're stronger and more capable now and ready to release more of the burden we've been carrying. We can move forward with even more grace and ease.

So, if this sounds like an adventure you'd like to be a part of, let's begin!

v. First Aid - If You Need To Shift NOW!

I realise that you might have picked up this book because your current situation is feeling unbearable, and you need something to shift now! Therefore, here are some First Aid tips which you can put into practice straight away. These will also help to lay a good foundation from which to launch your full wellbeing journey once you feel ready.

1. Explore my Self-Care Exercises playlist on YouTube (https://equenergy.com/SelfCareExercises). I mention these several times throughout this book as I strongly believe it's good to revisit them and to experiment to see which ones you resonate with and what works for you in the various situations you encounter. If you're feeling overwhelmed, I particularly recommend:

   * Collarbone Tapping
   * Breathing – Finger Tracing
   * Finger Holds
   * Getting outdoors into Nature

2. Read the section on Safety – see Chapter 3 p 87

3. A quick introduction to W·I·L·D®

W is for Wonder:

Pick an everyday object, such as a mug or a leaf. See if you can look at it with fresh eyes, as if you were a child, seeing it for the first time. How many 'wonder-full' things can you list about the object?

For the examples above, the mug might hold that wonderful first cuppa of the day, a warming drink when you come in from the cold, or something refreshing to quench your thirst on a hot day.

The leaf might be a crisp, vibrant green, or perhaps it's showing the changing colours of autumn. It might be an unusual shape with a delicate and intricate pattern of veins running through it.

Take at least 2 minutes each day to explore a new object and marvel at how it enriches your life.

I is for Intuition:

Take some time each day to sit in stillness and just listen to your body. Can you hear your breathing, your heart beating, or perhaps your digestion working away?

What can you feel - physically? emotionally?

What messages is your body sending you? Do you feel:
* tired or energised, hungry or thirsty
* any tightness or tension
* anxious or calm
* happy or sad, etc?

L is for Loving Yourself:

For this exercise, I invite you to imagine you're inviting yourself out on a date night. What might you do, where would you go, what would you like to chat about, and what might you say to your date?

How could you make yourself feel special, appreciated, and loved? What would this look like for you?

When you have a list, look through it and pick one 'date' each month and actually do this for yourself. Spend this time with you, getting to know yourself, your likes and dislikes and all your little idiosyncrasies. Give yourself permission to fall in love with the wonderful person who is You.

D is for Dance:

Dance is good for our bodies and good for our souls! This exercise involves listening to a variety of styles and tempos of music: classical, jazz, rock, rhythm & blues (R&B), folk and so on. Notice how you respond to each one, not just whether or not it's to your taste, but how you feel – physically and emotionally – when you listen to it. Feel into each piece and explore how your body might express it in movement. Then start to dance, feeling the rhythm, pace, mood and tone of each piece flowing through your body. Move with the music, go with its flow and see what it feels like to be in sync with it.

Bring in a sense of *Wonder*, letting your *Intuition* guide you as you explore your unique expression of the music, finding your personal relationship and harmony with it as you adapt to each style. *Lovingly* observe how you move and what this feels like for you. Remember there is no 'right' way to do this, and you can't get it 'wrong'. It's simply a form of explorative play, and the aim is to have fun and bring joy into the experience.

Now, explore how this practice of adapting to and flowing with the different pieces of music might support you in navigating the twists and turns of Life. What have you learnt about your physical, emotional and psychological flexibility? Can you draw on these learnings when facing challenges? What things change for you when you bring in a sense of fun and play?

Journal

With each of the exercises above, journal about what you felt and note any thoughts that came up and/or any insights you received. This will help deepen your self-awareness and emotional fluency.

From here, it's a matter of PPReLU:

Planning

- preparing for and deciding on the action you feel will best support you in shifting to a W·I·L·D® perspective and enhancing your self-care practice

Putting this action into Practice

Reviewing how you feel the practice went

- did you find it supportive/unsupportive, successful/unsuccessful and why?
- what did you learn about yourself, and what works for you?
- how has it expanded your knowledge of your body 'vocabulary' (how your body communicates with you through physical and emotional sensations)?
- what insights did you receive?

Learning from what you discovered in your review

- developing and growing your W·I·L·D® practice
- expanding your wellbeing toolkit

Updating your practice of W·I·L·D® from what you've learnt about yourself, your needs and your responses then repeat the process:

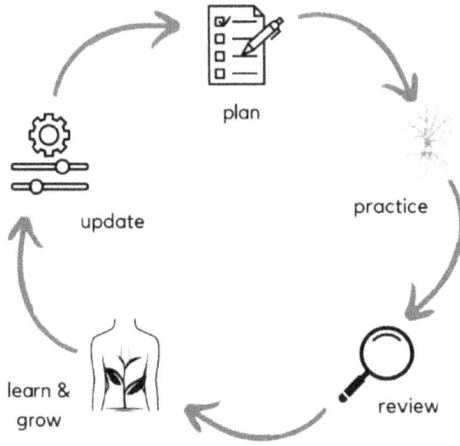

So, when you're ready, let's Take a Walk on the W·I·L·D® Side!

~ One ~
My Story ~ How it all Started

Inside Chapter One

Here, I share a bit about myself and my background to give you a sense of how my journey began. I hope you'll find aspects of my story relatable and realise I'm a regular human being, just like you. My aim is to give you the context behind the insights I've learnt, which I'll be sharing in this book, so you can get a deeper understanding of how they helped me and, in turn, how you might adopt and adapt them for yourself.

~ ~ ~ ~ ~

I would like to start this book with a 'pre-frame,' if I may. Parts of what I'll be sharing within these pages are raw and vulnerable and might, as such, be triggering for some readers; however, my intention is to illustrate that even when we feel at our lowest point, it is still possible to turn things around and to create the kind of life we long for.

Further, let me reassure you from the outset that there is a happy ending to my story despite its rather gloomy beginnings. In fact, my life now feels blessed with wonder and joy each and every day. My aim in sharing my story is to show you that reaching this happy ending is possible for you, too.

~ ~ ~ ~ ~

As I write this, I am fifty-five years of age – but there were times when I seriously doubted I'd ever make it this far. In my thirties, I was in a dark and unhappy place. I had reached the point of despair, feeling utterly hope-less and help-less[1]. Many times, I thought I couldn't go on. I didn't want to be here anymore; it was too painful. I just wanted the pain to end.

I tried everything I could think of to make things better - including going to my doctor, who put me on medication followed by counselling - but neither of these worked for me. I genuinely believed there was no way to make the pain stop, to the point where I would spend time thinking about and planning how I might end my life.

If you've ever been there yourself, I hear you. If you know someone who has, I feel you. It is a lonely and desperate place. So, what changed for me if I am here writing this book?

In short, I've known several people who chose to end their lives, including a friend, two work colleagues and the one who undoubtedly had the most impact, my dad. I've seen the pain their actions left behind, and I couldn't bear the thought of doing this to my family. I figured it would be better for me to suffer myself than to inflict such immense pain on the people I loved.

There is such a lot packed within that last sentence. For a start, there's the fact that I believed my feelings mattered less than anyone else's. Looking back, this is hugely revealing because it shows just how I saw myself at that time. In fact, years later, when I started on my journey of Meta Consciousness®[2] , the initial report I received from my practitioner noted that my self-esteem was 'severely damaged'. Then there's the immense feelings of guilt, pain, and even anger I experienced following each person's death — especially that of my dad. I questioned:

- Why did they do it?
- Why did they not talk to me about how they were feeling?

---

1   Throughout this book you'll see there are some words that I divide in this way (e.g., hope-less, power-full, dis-ease, in-joy, bio-logical). Words (and what we say – particularly to ourselves) are very significant and hold a creative energy. What we think or say repeatedly, becomes true for us. Also, how we relate to the words, and the meaning we give them, is critical. Dividing the words in this way gives them a new and more profound impact for me, and changes how I relate to them. If this doesn't feel the same for you then don't worry. You can still read the words as you normally would and be reassured that the content of this book will not be affected.
2   I will be discussing this in much more depth later in this book.

- How could I not notice/understand how unhappy they were?
- Could I have done more to support them?
- How could they leave me in such a hurtful way?

Even when our heads might be able to rationalise what's happened, our hearts are still reeling with the intense emotion of it all. This meant that my head was full of possible opportunities I might have missed, along with the 'why's' and 'what if's' that would now never be answered.

If I focus on the passing of my dad, I was left wondering where this left me. How did I cope with the loss? How did I cope with the guilt and feeling that I should have done more? How did I manage my feelings when I wasn't even able to fully acknowledge them?

Thankfully, my inner stubborn streak came out – a trait which won't allow me to be a 'quitter' - and it reminded me in no uncertain terms that I couldn't take the same path (for all the reasons I've mentioned). It would be unfair on those left behind and wouldn't achieve anything except for more pain, so, after much soul searching, I decided that I didn't want to be defined by what had happened and that I no longer wanted to live this grey shadow of a life.

This realisation was so profound that it prompted me to set out on a journey, and it is this journey that I will be sharing with you right here in this book. I hope that if you, too, are feeling lost, help-less and alone, I can (through the medium of my words) shine a light into that darkness and help you to believe that there is hope. Not only that but there is the potential for a brighter future. If you can trust enough to ask in your heart – or even cry out if you need to - you will start to see that the answers are there for you to find.

Throughout these pages, I will be sharing what has enabled me to go from being someone who *felt*:

- useless
- ugly
- unworthy

- not good enough
- small
- unwanted
- unlovable

To becoming someone who *knows* that:

- These are just feelings – they're not Who I Really Am.

You will learn:

- I'd been responding to beliefs formed due to early experiences and conditioning, which had limited me and caused me to shut down parts of myself—but these beliefs weren't serving me.
- How I put these aside – and how you can too – in order to step into the fullness of our True Nature[1].
- How I came to understand that my feelings and symptoms held rich wisdom, and it was this wisdom that I used to navigate my way back to wellbeing. I also achieved a greater sense of comfort within my own skin – and you hold the ability for your body to achieve this, too.
- How I finally realised that my body wasn't going wrong/attacking me/betraying me/letting me down, and that I wasn't ugly. In fact, I was able to reframe those thoughts and acknowledge that my body is this most amazing, intelligent system that does SO many wonderful things for me every day – and you will learn how to acknowledge this, too. Everything that was true for me is equally true for you.

I am now happier and healthier than I've ever been.

I no longer suffer from IBS (irritable bowel syndrome)[2], eczema,

---

1   By 'True Nature' I mean the real you, underneath any conditioning or baggage that you might have accumulated during your lifetime. It's the person you were born to be, when you are free to share all the wonderful gifts that are uniquely yours.
2   "Irritable bowel syndrome is a 'disorder of gut-brain interaction' characterized by a group of symptoms that commonly include abdominal pain and or abdominal bloating and changes in the consistency of bowel movements. These symptoms may occur over a long time, sometime's for years." (https://en.wikipedia.org/wiki/Irritable_bowel_syndrome)

migraines or chronic fatigue. The anxiety and depression that used to fill my days have greatly reduced, AND whilst they occasionally still rear their head, I now see these moments as information – thoughts that I can sit down and dialogue with out of curiosity and then go on to address with compassion.

If you're reading this and thinking something along the lines of, *'That's all very well for you, but I could never get to that point. I don't have the strength/skills/brains/money/support/time/ or whatever to do this…'*, then I need to let you know that there is absolutely nothing special about me. I, too, had those same thoughts – they're what held me stuck for so long - but through my journey, I've come to understand where these thoughts come from and that they are actually part of the whole process – there's a reason for them. It's not – as I'd previously thought – that there was something wrong with me or that I was lacking something everyone around me seemed to have; it was just that I was carrying all kinds of unhelpful beliefs. As *Abraham-Hicks*[1] once said:

"A belief is just a thought you keep thinking."

Beliefs are thoughts. They are not truths about me. And they're not truths about you either.

Remember – there is a reason for all of our thoughts, and they are the backbone of our healing journey. Once we understand their purpose, we can embrace them and begin to use them for good.

I understand this can be tough to get your head around but trust me, whatever negative thoughts you have about yourself are not true, any more than the thoughts I had about myself were.

But why should you trust me on this?

As you read through this book, you will learn more about my story, which, I hope, will help you to see that if someone like *me* can change my life for the better, then it is absolutely possible for you to do so.

---

1   https://www.abraham-hicks.com/

When you begin to see your own results, you'll realise that you no longer need to trust me because now you are trusting yourself.

To begin, I mentioned in the opening few sentences that I was feeling utterly miserable, hope-less and help-less and that medication and counselling weren't working for me. Don't get me wrong, both can be hugely beneficial, but using these and their subsequent success depends on several factors, not least of which is you yourself, your situation and, of course, which doctors and/or counsellors you connect with.

For me I was approaching these remedies in the early 2000s, and I know that practices have changed extensively since then. It is entirely possible that if I were using these now, I would experience a different outcome, so I would never suggest not trying these avenues if they feel appropriate for you. There is **absolutely** a place for medication and therapies; I am simply offering you the chance to explore complementary approaches based on my own experiences, knowledge and research.

Once these avenues (medication and counselling) proved ineffective, it felt as if they were essentially 'closed', so I was once again lost with nowhere to turn. As far as I was concerned, I'd tried everything, and nothing was working, but I genuinely felt there had to be some kind of solution. In the end, being a bit of a bookworm, I decided to do some reading.

Growing up in the '80s, I was familiar with the concept of the *Self Help Book*, and because we were yet to enjoy the benefits of the internet, I went off to the library in search of answers within the pages of these books.

Reading up on something with which I was already familiar seemed a good place to begin, so I read Neale Donald Walsch's, '*Conversations with God*' trilogy. This might seem an odd starting point, but I was brought up as a Catholic in Northern Ireland in the 1970s, which meant that religion had always been a big part of my life.

I felt drawn to faith and spirituality, to the idea of something bigger than myself, and to a force of Life, Love and Growth behind this Universe in which we live, so I thought it would be a good place to explore initially. Though I often struggled with the conflicts between, and even within, faiths along with their inconsistencies and contradictions, I still felt drawn to Walsch's trilogy, so this is where I began.

When I read *'Conversations with God'*, it was the first time I encountered the concept of Love being at our core[1] (which he refers to as 'Who I Really Am'). Walsch went on to state that many of us are not currently living from this place, and as someone who had been feeling ugly, unwanted, and deeply different from those around me, I began to wonder if this was true for me. Did I have Love at the core of my being? And actually, if I doubted this, if I chose not to believe I have Love at the core of my being, was this, in fact, a form of arrogance? Did I somehow think I was special and different from everyone else, that for some reason, this rule – having Love at the core of my being - did not apply to me? This was an uncomfortable train of thought as I was brought up believing arrogance to be a 'mortal sin', so I was left with two opposing ideas:

1. that I was displaying traits of arrogance in daring to believe I was different to everyone else so methods which worked for them would not work for me.
2. that I didn't have Love at my core and had no idea how to achieve this.

The more I read, the more I became aware of cognitive dissonance (lack of harmony), and I didn't know which was true: what I *believed* about myself or what I was *reading*. The first left me feeling deeply unhappy, yet the second felt completely out of my reach.

It wasn't long before I became fascinated by the concept that perhaps there was this hidden core within me that actually IS Love, is beautiful,

---

1   If it's true that my core is Love, then when I live from this place, everything I do is done with the highest of vibrations: love, compassion and joy. However, when I'm not living from this place my actions are coloured by less uplifting emotions such as bitterness, jealousy, fear and rage (see the Emotion Scale in Appendix 3).

and is exactly as I was designed to be. If this were true, it would mean I wasn't broken, ugly, unlovable, or unworthy, so I expanded this thought. Could I find this part of me and get to know her? Could I start living from this place of Love rather than from a place of negativity and despair?

This is ultimately the question that led to this book, albeit many years later, but in order for you to continue on this journey with me, I need to add some context. Why did I carry such negative beliefs, and why did I believe that I was ugly, broken, and unlovable?

To find the answers, we need to go back to the very beginning.

The early years

I was born in Belfast in 1968, the first of two children – a brother was to follow. My mum came from a large family of seven, and my dad came from a family of four. I always knew that Mum had hoped for a large family herself, but, due to experiencing several miscarriages, in the end, there was just me and my brother.

Religion was such a divisive issue in Northern Ireland at that time and was blamed for many of the country's struggles. Mum's family are

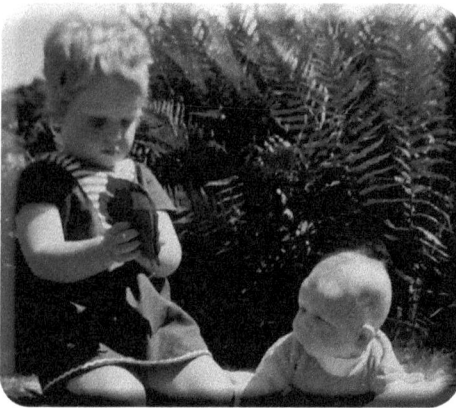

Catholic, and Dad's Presbyterian, though he had converted to Catholicism before I came along. We lived on the east side of the city, away from the worst of the violence and division; however, it remained a constant backdrop to my childhood. I still remember, when I was about seven years old, realising that the country was founded on two opposing sides and religions, which caused considerable hurt and unrest. I felt foolish that I hadn't noticed it earlier – even though I was still only a child – because it was (and to an extent remains) such a big issue within

Ireland. To my childhood brain, it made little sense, and I remember thinking that the adults were crazy for creating and perpetuating all this unnecessary – to me - antagonism and hatred. After all, we were the same people, living in the same country – geographically, at least, if not politically. Growing up as a Catholic in this era of 'The Troubles' meant I felt part of an unwanted and sometimes despised minority.

('The Troubles' refers to the violence and division within the Northern Irish community between the Loyalists - mostly Protestant people who support the right of the British Government to rule the province - and the Republicans - mostly Catholics who view the British as colonisers and who would advocate for Ireland to be reunited as one country under their own rule. 'The Troubles' first erupted in 1968 due to unrest following a Civil Rights march and then escalated into bombings, shootings, abductions and open aggression between communities. The British Army were brought in to keep the peace but in fact the situation only deteriorated further following their arrival. Each side was fuelled by anger, bitterness, hatred and distrust. People stayed within their own communities and generally – with only a few notable exceptions - did not mix with each other. Everyone lived within a background of fear but as Catholics were in the minority, they often felt that life was particularly unfair for members of their community. One example of this is when the Protestant Orange Parades demanded the right to march along Catholic streets. Catholics saw this as a Protestant show of strength and dominance, which was therefore deeply resented.)

Added to this and within my own family, I remember feeling that I was a 'nuisance' and that I should have been born a boy. My dad would chastise me for being 'too sensitive' and would shout comments such as, *'Stop crying, or I'll give you something to cry about'*. I found this deeply confusing. If my dad 'gave me something to cry about', surely I would just cry more? But then you're already angry with me, so won't that make it worse?

My brother arrived in 1971, and I instantly felt that he was more loved and accepted simply because he was a boy. I don't mind admitting I was jealous of him.

Their increased love and acceptance of him (as perceived by me) could have been purely because he was a baby and depended entirely on my parents, but at the same time, I also remember being expected to be the responsible one and to look after my brother when, at three years old, I didn't even feel able to take care of myself. If I wasn't able to get things 'right' myself, how could I possibly make my infant brother do so? This led, inevitably, to me being blamed not just for my mistakes but for his as well.

I've also since learnt that I was a colicky baby and cried a lot, so Dad 'banished' me to the bedroom furthest from theirs, which is an interesting point to consider. As a baby, I would have been too young to be aware of this and attach any significance to it, but did I subconsciously feel unwanted and did that message follow me through life?

Mum has also told me in later years that both she and dad would scold me without any issue, but they rarely told me when I had done well. She said that they would tell me off when things went wrong but didn't know how to balance this out with praise. Consequently, I grew up being afraid to even try most of the time, as I expected to fail and be punished no matter what I did. The message I received was that nothing ever seemed to be good enough, which I interpreted as *'I'm not good enough'*.

Interestingly, looking back now, I can see that my dad was sometimes reluctant to do things himself because he didn't want to be seen to 'fail'. If he hadn't learnt how to navigate this himself, it follows that he wouldn't have been able to pass on this skill either.

In more recent years, I've followed the work of *Dr Gabor Maté* who talks a lot about 'trauma'. According to this well-regarded Canadian physician, 'trauma' doesn't just relate to obvious examples, such as being in a multi-car pile-up, witnessing something like the dreadful Twin Towers disaster of 9/11, or having a serious, life-changing accident. Instead, he says that:

*"Trauma isn't what happens to you. It's what happens **inside** you as a result of what happens **to** you."*

He goes on to explain that trauma is actually a sense of disconnection, or as Stephen Porges (an American psychologist) puts it, 'a chronic disruption of connection'. So, if a child experiences a sense of disconnection from their caregiver(s), which, for some reason, isn't then repaired, this can be traumatising for them.

Studies[1] have shown that if a mother is depressed, her child is much more likely to develop certain traits such as anxiety and hypervigilance. Dr Maté reasons that a depressed mother may be preoccupied with her worries and is, therefore, less able to be emotionally present, grounded and balanced for her infant. The sensitive child will pick up on this and experience the same feelings as their mother, but, as they are an infant, they haven't yet developed the ability to regulate their own inner systems or to process these strong emotions, so they feel overwhelmed. The only option they have in the face of this pain, therefore, (and without the support they need to process it) is to shut down.

This isn't a conscious choice. It's a survival strategy—and it works. The baby lives and grows up through childhood, adolescence, and adulthood. However—and this is where the problem can really manifest—if they haven't learnt more appropriate coping strategies during this time, they (as adults) can continue to shut down, tune out, or run away from things they find overwhelming and scary.

Think about that for a moment. What we learn as babies – even if we are unaware– will stay with us throughout our lives and shape our beliefs as adults, BUT because we learn them as children, we do not have the tools to manage them as adults.

Learning this suddenly made so much sense to me. Over the last few years, Mum has shared bits and pieces about her own experiences growing up and what happened whilst she was married to my dad. She herself was experiencing a lot of deeply challenging issues at a time when she was far away from 'home' (i.e., the town where she grew up) and found herself without any form of support network. Her own mum

---

1   As detailed in the work of Gabor Maté. See references at the end of the book.

had died when she was a teenager and, as the eldest of five siblings, mum had taken on much of the care of her younger brother and sisters. Her father then remarried and had two more children.

Mum went away to university before returning to Ireland and then moved from the familiarity of her home town to Belfast for work. She met my dad through mutual friends, and he appeared to be a charming young man. They got engaged and married – then he changed. Overnight. In fact, years later and after his death, Mum described Dad's behaviour to a specialist and was told that he had shown definite signs of schizoid[2] tendencies.

It was a very difficult, lonely and stressful time for Mum, with my dad often out of work, the miscarriages she experienced, and then having two young children to raise with no day-to-day support either from her husband or her family (who were about an hour and a half drive away). The more I learnt about my parents, the more I realised how much my upbringing had impacted my perception of Self[3], and it is entirely possible that the same is true for you.

It is not my intention to point fingers of blame, and, having done a lot of work on this, I am no longer looking for the sympathy I once craved. I have come to understand that **everyone in my life was doing the very best they could with the resources they had available to them and with the beliefs that they held.**

And really, they could do no more because they simply didn't have the tools, learnings, structures, opportunities, support, etc. to do so.

I mentioned above that my parents would scold me when I did something wrong and wouldn't balance this out with praise for the things I did right. Nowadays, slapping children is frowned upon, but

---

2 'Schizoid tendencies' – I've never been able to get to the bottom of what this actually means but it seems that my dad might have been showing behaviours that could have indicated schizophrenia or a schizotypal personality disorder (i.e. 'odd or eccentric behaviour, social withdrawal, paranoid or bizarre ideas not amounting to true delusions, thought disorder and perceptual disturbances' https://www.therecoveryvillage.com/mental-health/schizotypal-personality-disorder/)
3 That is, of who we are. Often, we tend to focus on the aspects of our identity that relate to our roles, such as teacher, mother, doctor, father, brother, etc. Here I'm thinking more about how we perceive ourselves and our place in the world aside from these labels.

when I was growing up, it was quite normal and seen as the way to instil good discipline. At the time, discipline was considered to be the root of responsible parenting; thus, mine were just doing the best they knew, given the tools they had at the time. They simply wanted to teach me 'right from wrong', keep me safe and help me navigate the world in which we lived.

Parenting methods when I was a child differed hugely in other ways, too. In the 1960s and 70s, new parents were often told that if their baby cried when it was put to bed, then it should be left to cry. It was believed that going back to soothe it was 'mollycoddling' (being indulgent or over-protective) and would teach the child that it could manipulate its parents in order to get its own way. Today (2024), it is no longer considered the best approach to leave a baby to cry. In the same way that the toddler 'naughty step' principle is not as commonly used as it once was.

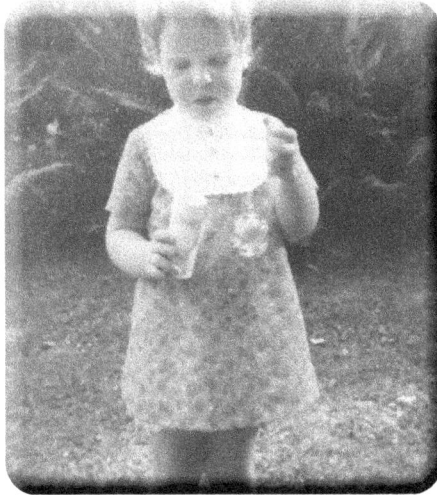

Childrearing methods change as we learn more about the impact they have on the development of the infant, its brain and internal systems, and we need to remember, too, that our parents are largely the product of their *own* upbringing. It is possible that my mum and dad didn't praise me because this wasn't something they themselves experienced. Similarly, they might have been (overly) strict because their parents were too. When I reflect, I can rationalise that it wasn't only my parents who were this way; I experienced exactly the same at school, in church and when visiting some of my friends too.

In fact, I want to acknowledge here that my mum did an amazing job. She worked, she looked after the house, and she took care of me and my brother. When we were young, she would take long holidays over the summer, and although we didn't have much money, she came up with wonderful, creative games for us to play and took us on interesting trips. We'd go out into Nature[4] and visit museums, for example. These are my happy memories.

When Dad was around, though, things were different. He was the one whose attention I craved, and I remember idolising him when I was small. Perhaps this was because I desperately wanted a sense of attachment. I wanted to feel important to him, safe and cared for. I wanted to have a great relationship with him and to feel that he loved me. I was always trying to get on his good side and often believed I fell short. His moods were volatile, and instead of feeling safe and loved, I lived on a knife edge, wanting his approval but fearing his temper. I think all three of us – Mum, my brother and I – walked on eggshells around him. Later, I was to discover that he was a functioning alcoholic – he could drink and not appear to get drunk – which undoubtedly had an impact.

As a child, I was shielded from this. I didn't know or understand what was going on with him, yet I instinctively felt that he wasn't happy, and I longed to change this. Even then, I could sense there was a potential for something better for him, for a better life if the unhappiness inside of him could be addressed. I continued to try to uplift his mood, even though I had no experience or reference; I just felt that I wanted to make him cheerful. In the end, Mum reached the point where she could no longer accept my dad's behaviour. In addition to being an alcoholic, it transpired that he had indulged in several affairs, and one day, Mum told him to leave. I was thirteen at this point, and my brother was ten. It was a huge shock and I genuinely hadn't seen it coming. Despite the fact that I knew my parents weren't happy, Irish Catholics – and our family in particular - didn't get divorced, certainly not in my experience. It was a bolt out of the blue and hit me hard.

---

4   *I often write Nature with a capital 'N' as I think of her like Mother Nature, a guiding, supporting, nurturing force in our lives.*

Dad called a family meeting to tell us he was going. We'd never had a family meeting before. He said (at least this is what I heard and how I remember it) that my brother would be okay because he was Mum's favourite, and I'd be okay as I was a loner like him. All I could think was, *'Just goes to show how little you know me'* (for I wasn't a loner) and *'So it's true then – my brother is the favourite!'*

On the surface, though, he was partly right. I was a loner, but only because I struggled to make friends. I found it hard to connect with my peers and to relax into the flow of playground interactions. I would get deeply hurt and feel rejected by the shift of friendships that is normal amongst young children. I hadn't developed the resilience and flexibility required, and, as a result, I found myself on my own—a lot.

The next few years were challenging. Mum tried to maintain a connection between Dad, my brother and myself, but he didn't make this easy, often cancelling at the last minute or just not showing up. I hated and resented these arrangements and subsequent let-downs, but I didn't feel able to speak up or express how I felt.

My world became unstable and unpredictable, which added to my stress levels, and it was during this time that I first started to experience migraines and IBS[5].

Then, when I was sixteen years old, I got glandular fever. The timing wasn't great, but I was determined not to miss too much school because if I did, I would have to re-sit the whole year and leave behind the people I knew. I would have to start again with a new bunch of people, which I would find hard. The thought of such a change terrified me, so I pushed myself to return to school before I fully recovered. In the end, I couldn't cope and had to re-sit the year anyway.Going back a year tapped into my 'failure' mentality, and I felt totally lost and alone. The stress mounted; I wasn't eating properly and lost a lot of weight, eventually dropping to 4.5 stone (63lb / 28.6kg). This resulted in me ending up in hospital where they initially diagnosed anorexia, though later changed this to depression. All I knew was that I was

---

5   *See previous note about Irritable Bowel Syndrome*

deeply unhappy and didn't care about myself. In fact, I would go as far as to say there were elements of self-loathing and punishment along with a need for control, both of which manifested in my behaviours at the time.

I'd love to be able to say this experience prompted me to address the pain I held inside, enabling me to make positive changes and move forward with my life, but to be honest, I think I simply exchanged one form of control and avoidance for another. After leaving the hospital, my relationship with my body and with food were no better, but I made myself eat so that I wouldn't have to go through the shame of being hospitalised a second time. I also didn't want to ever upset Mum so deeply again.

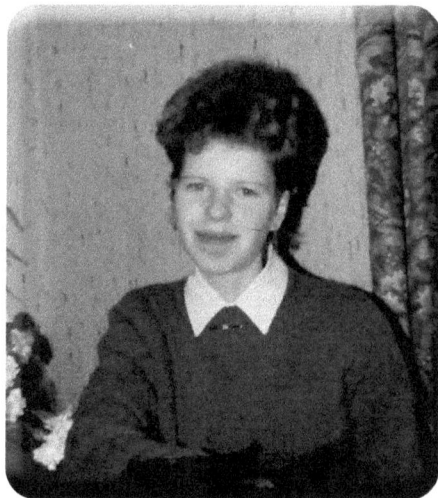

During all of this, I still believed that I was a broken, ugly person and continued to punish myself as a way to avoid looking at how deeply I was hurting. It wasn't a conscious decision; it was just a learnt behaviour. I didn't have the words to express how I felt - I didn't even know where to begin. All I knew was how to grit my teeth and carry on; there was no other option (known in my family as 'G&B' – 'grin and bear it').

Despite these challenges, I was still expected to study hard, finish school and go to a good university – so I did. I chose to go to Manchester to train as a Teacher for the Deaf. I'd been learning British Sign Language since I was about sixteen and had spent a lot of time in the Deaf Community in Belfast, so it seemed like a logical step.

At first, I was dreadfully homesick, but then I began to really enjoy my independence. I was settling in and enjoying my studies – and then I was dealt another blow. I got sick again. This time, it was an inner ear infection which resulted in debilitating vertigo, and I ended up having to leave my course and return home. From there, my condition deteriorated. Before long, I found myself in a wheelchair and then eventually confined to bed.

Medical advice was sought, and even though it took a long time, I was finally diagnosed with myalgic encephalomyelitis (ME), which, at this time (the late 1980's) wasn't recognised by mainstream medicine and was referred to as 'yuppie flu'. As a result, the only support - and even understanding - I received came from good friends and complementary approaches. With little choice, I was forced to rest a lot, which led to me finding new ways of expressing how I was feeling - through drawing - and I know having this outlet really supported my eventual recovery. Mum was absolutely amazing. For a start, she never once questioned my illness or doubted that it was real – unlike the doctors. She also refused to give up searching for ways to help me heal, and that was how I first discovered the world of complementary therapies - and where I finally received an understanding and recognition of my condition.

ME, for me, manifested as deep fatigue and aches and pains throughout my body. I also experienced poor memory and debilitating brain fog. I often felt nauseated, and my head would ache. I just wanted to sleep and had no energy or interest in anything.

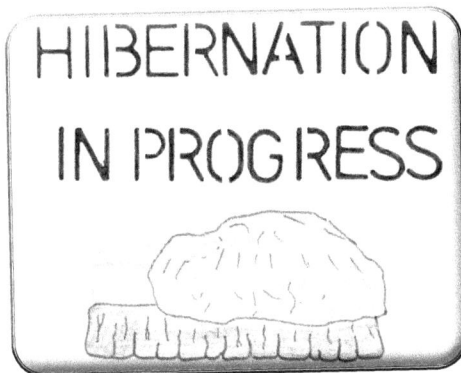

HIBERNATION
IN PROGRESS

Some days, I would feel a little better, but any activity or the slightest stress would cause my symptoms to return. ME is also sometimes referred to as Post Viral Fatigue Syndrome, which speaks to the belief that I developed it as a result of the glandular fever I'd had years before. I was about twenty years old when the ME was eventually diagnosed, so I had been unwell in some form or other for about four years.

I often say that, in many ways, my illness was much worse for Mum. She watched my health go downhill, unable to do anything to help, and she must have been acutely aware of all that I was missing out on. For me, I just withdrew and slept. It was a strange space where time seemed to stand still whilst everyone else carried on moving forward. My peers were out having fun, exploring life and making choices for their future, but this wasn't something I felt able to do. Consequently, I think I missed out on a lot of the learning and personal development that comes from this kind of socialising.

During this time, I remember reading a book (sadly, I can't remember what it was called), which brought me to a profound realisation: how I'd been feeling – the fatigue, brain fog, aches, and so on – had been *serving a purpose* for me. With the language I've learnt now, I can reflect on these symptoms and say they had become an adaptation my body originally made in order to help me survive a really painful and challenging time in my life. When life had felt too big, overwhelming, complex and even threatening, my body had slipped further and further into the strategy it had learnt early on – to shut down, withdraw and retreat.

These adaptations that our bodies make are subconscious, but reading this book helped me to understand that (a) the adaptations existed and (b) they were no longer serving me well. What had manifested in childhood as a feeling of failure and inadequacy was now showing itself as various ills.

Though I didn't yet know how to, this was the start of me realising I had (some form of) control over my body and that it was down to me to put aside the fearful beliefs and make the decision to start living again. This, I believed, greatly supported my recovery from ME.

The next couple of years were some of the happiest of my life. I was in my early twenties, I had a job I loved (working at a church for Deaf people), and an amazing boss. I also had friends and a social life, and at last felt like I was finding my direction and purpose.

After a while, this purpose began to develop into a calling. Faith, as I said, has always been a big part of my life, and so I started to consider dedicating my life to it. I researched joining a convent and actually went to stay in one in County Mayo for a month's trial. At the time I believed this route was exactly the one for me.

Unfortunately, whilst I was away, I received a phone call to tell me that my dad had collapsed and been rushed to hospital. He was seriously ill. I remember walking out into the convent gardens and becoming lost in my thoughts. It was a beautiful spring day; the skylarks were hovering and calling … and suddenly, I knew with absolute certainty that Dad had died. A couple of minutes later, one of the nuns appeared. Dad had indeed died.

The nuns were incredibly kind and arranged transport for me to return to Belfast. Though I had no way of knowing, that was the last time I was to be a part of the life of that convent.

Once home, the next few days passed in a blur as details emerged about how Dad had died and arrangements were made for his funeral. I found out that the neighbours who lived below had heard a thud, seen Dad's milk bottles still outside the door and called the police, who broke down the door. Dad had collapsed in the bathroom. He was rushed to hospital, but it was too late. His organs were already shutting down, and despite their best efforts, Dad could not be saved.

From then on, it became like a kind of crazy soap opera. The police remained involved because they found things in Dad's flat, which made them suspicious of paramilitary connections. I was struggling to cope, particularly when I looked into the bathroom and saw where the police had drawn around Dad's false teeth. They must have come out of his mouth when he collapsed, which left his bathroom looking like something from a TV crime drama. This image stayed with me for many years, and I could feel its physical impact any time I saw or heard about a similar situation.

I also discovered that there had been a rather awkward moment at the hospital. Mum, along with Dad's girlfriend, arrived at the same time, and the hospital staff couldn't get their heads around who was who and why they had arrived together. For my part, I was in pieces. Mum, my brother and I went to Dad's flat - Mum was determined to clean it (it was in a terrible state) – even though there was no onus on her to do so. But I guess that was her way of coping with this unthinkable situation. Mum sent me out to buy some flowers, and I ended up sitting on a wall by the sea in the town where Dad had lived. Looking out over the ocean, I cried as if my heart would break.

You may wonder at my reaction when, as I've previously mentioned, my relationship with Dad was, at times, toxic and negative. The thing is, grief is incredibly complex and can be very challenging to navigate. We can find ourselves going through a rollercoaster of emotions all within one day or even a matter of minutes. It isn't a linear process either, meaning it can bring up several emotions at once rather than one after another and bring us back to feelings we thought we'd dealt with. In addition to the sadness of our loss, guilt and shame are often common. My grief at Dad's death was, therefore, compounded by the mixed-up emotions I had around our relationship. I'd always loved him – he was my dad, after all – and felt deep empathy for his pain, but I was angry and experienced betrayal by him, too.

I'd wanted him to be a loving father who supported me and cared about me, but I never felt this. Instead, he left me with unanswered questions, anxiety and confusion.

I went through the funeral in a daze. It was a cremation, which felt as if we were on a conveyor belt: in, short service led by someone who knew nothing about Dad; out again by another door as the next family arrived; and finally, trying to pick out which flowers were ours amongst all the bouquets and wreaths propped against the wall. I was numb with grief and didn't feel able to express my pain in front of Mum and her family (who never really got on with my dad).

Dad's family was represented by his two sisters, but they didn't even come over to speak to us. The only person from Dad's side who acknowledged us was a man who looked vaguely familiar, though I couldn't place him. It turned out he was someone I used to see at a bus stop years earlier when I was on my way to work each morning. He had a little dog, and we'd got chatting. Often, he would call "Hello!" as I walked past. Seeing him at Dad's funeral was surreal, but in this strange world of coincidences, he told me that he'd actually gone to school with my dad, which is something neither of us knew before that hideous day. Having a virtual stranger with us to say goodbye was odd but a small comfort nonetheless, particularly as he remembered me and had taken the time to come over and speak with us.

Over the next few weeks, I slowly returned to something resembling normal life, but I was still carrying my grief deep inside. No one else seemed to feel the same way, though, so I pushed it down, thinking that somehow it was a betrayal to express it. I couldn't make sense of my emotions, given my complicated relationship with my dad, and when others appeared to handle it with ease, I felt even more of an outsider. That child who was 'getting it wrong' again.

When the inquest into Dad's death ended, things became even more challenging. The coroner concluded that Dad had died due to a combination of alcohol and pills. Effectively, according to the coroner, Dad had made the decision to leave us. Apparently, he had been storing up his medication, which he then took all at once - which is what caused his organs to fail. This hurt my mum, my brother and myself deeply. I felt he had robbed us of the opportunity to understand why he had done this or, indeed, understand some of the things we had experienced with him over the years. I didn't know how to handle so many conflicting emotions; they felt overwhelming, too heavy a burden to carry, particularly as there was no one I could talk to.

I was riddled with guilt. Dad and I had been to Donegal together a few months before, and I'd suspected something was wrong at the time as he had hardly spoken. The trip had been excruciating, and all I could think was how uncomfortable it had been for me.

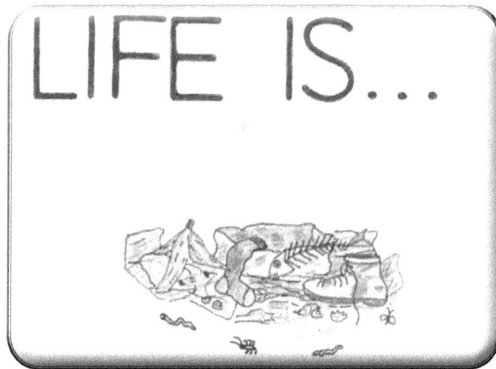

LIFE IS...

With hindsight, I wondered if I had been selfish and blind. I hadn't been there on the day dad had died, and I hadn't picked up on any of the signs pointing to how seriously unwell he was. If I had taken the time to reach out, might things have taken a different course? This was a question which tortured me endlessly. Then, I would rationalise and realise that even if I had tried, I would have feared making him angry – so perhaps I wouldn't have done anything differently.

Following Dad's death and funeral, my plan had been to go back to the convent, but I was told I couldn't return until I had first undertaken some counselling. The Church found a therapist for me in Belfast, and I started going along for weekly sessions. Rather than helping, though, I found it incredibly traumatising. The woman insisted on calling me 'Miss Palmer', which I hated – it felt so formal and distant - and I remember having to lie on a bed in a room in her house which had rainbow wallpaper. It must have been a kid's bedroom, which was a complete mismatch for this formal, painful experience. The therapist would sit quietly behind me and wait for me to talk, yet I didn't know what to say. I dreaded each session and would spend the entire bus journey trying to think of things to talk about during my upcoming meeting.

Interestingly, I've since learnt that to experience healing, we need to feel completely safe and connected. I didn't feel this at all, so it's no wonder this particular therapy didn't work for me.

I continued to go along, though, knowing it was expected of me, until one day, something suddenly clicked, and I realised I could make a choice.

I could stop going to counselling. I didn't have to keep turning up.

Such a momentous choice would mean I wouldn't be able to return to the convent as I wouldn't have completed the required counselling, but if this kind of counselling was something they insisted upon, then perhaps becoming a nun was not the right vocation for me.

This was the first time I allowed myself to listen to my gut - my True Nature – and let it guide me. Decision made. At the very next appointment, I told the therapist I wouldn't be coming back. She appeared to take this as a sign that the counselling was working and tried to insist I carry on, but I stuck to my decision and left.

On reflection, the counselling had worked in some way, even if only to help me realise this approach was not right for me. Travelling home on the bus that final day, I felt a sense of lightness and liberation. The moment was deeply empowering and is something I still think back to if I need to remind myself how power-full it can feel to listen to my heart and to follow what I know on a deep level, is right for me.

With my career path now changed, I was fortunate to get a job where I'd worked before and slotted back into my 'old' life with relative ease. The contract was only temporary, though, and my boss, looking ahead, encouraged me to further my qualifications as a way to support my career. By this stage, I was also doing some sign language interpreting work, both within the church and at the local further education college, so he suggested I take a formal course in this field. It meant going to England to study, but I grabbed the chance with both hands and ended up in Bristol, where I earned a Diploma in Deaf Studies.

The tutors there were amazing, top people in their field, which meant the teaching was at a very high standard. Unfortunately, two particular tutors, whilst highly skilled and respected, did not seem able to nurture and encourage their students, which left most of our cohort feeling demotivated. This experience echoed back to my past when, as a child, I had been corrected when I had done something wrong but never encouraged when I had done something well.

It was during my time in Bristol that I met someone who I fell in love with, and a while later, we got engaged. After finishing my studies, I secured a job in Kent (working as a sign language interpreter in a multi-disciplinary team), so my fiancé and I moved there to live. (Luckily, he was able to secure a career transfer to Dartford).We married in September 1995, and I tried hard to settle into my new life in Kent, but my job was stressful, even within our lovely small interpreting team, and neither my husband nor I really made any friends in the area. Then, suddenly, his father died. We returned to Bristol for the funeral, and when we got back to our flat in Kent, I received a letter informing me that a job had arisen at the university department in Bristol, where I had studied. My husband and I considered our options and decided that I would apply for the job, and if successful, we would consider moving back to Bristol to be near his mum and friends. I passed the interview and secured the job, and within a few months, we were back in Bristol and looking to buy a house - however, our marriage was not going well.

It had been a stressful time; our jobs were challenging, and neither of us were able to communicate how we were feeling, so we simply stopped supporting ourselves and each other. Inevitably, things began to fall apart.

One morning, I remember sitting on my own downstairs, and I literally felt something in my chest, almost as if my heart had broken. I knew then that I couldn't carry on this way. I told my husband that I wanted a divorce.

Even though I had been the one to initiate the process, it was one of the most painful things I have ever experienced. I asked myself countless times how I could do something so hurtful to my husband. He didn't take it well either and called me many unkind and cruel names. It really shook my sense of Self; even though I understood his reaction, I knew that I needed to do this for my own sanity. Further, I hated that I was repeating the pattern set by my parents, and, on reflection, if I'd had a better set of tools, perhaps I could have handled things differently, or at least in a better way, but sadly, I didn't have that skill set.

Around the same time, I met a man who gave me a glimpse of what a better relationship could look like, how it might feel to have fun in my life again and to know that I was a human being rather than someone who simply worked, looked after the house and acted as a personal taxi driver. Slowly, this relationship helped me to recover from the pain of my divorce, and I started to enjoy a normal social life again - even though work continued to be stressful. After a while, we moved in together, and life seemed to be looking up – until the year 2000. That's when I began to really struggle in my role at the university.

For a long time, my boss had been demonstrating behaviour which could be classed as bullying, and I found this incredibly triggering because it reminded me of my relationship with my dad. Alongside the bullying, my role had become increasingly demanding with little to no additional support, and, due to funding issues, I was issued with my P45 every month until the money for another four weeks' salary was confirmed. This went on month after month after month until, in the end (and after a helpful comment from my partner suggesting I'd had a 'sense of humour bypass'), I realised I couldn't do this anymore. I handed in my notice and went freelance.

Though I still ended up working mostly at the university, now it was on my terms, and I could walk away at the end of each assignment.

In 2005, my partner and I married, and a year later, his son moved in with us. Though he's a wonderful young man, suddenly having a 16-year-old living with us was difficult to navigate as both my husband and I had very different perspectives. My husband was quite laid back, yet I wanted clarity on my role and my boundaries as a 'stepmother' who had never parented before. My husband, for example, worked shifts at the time, and I didn't know if he was happy for his son to bring a girl back to the house. And if so, was she allowed to stay over? Unfortunately, the less supported I felt, the more I needed clarity. I didn't feel 'safe' and retreated into my own headspace, detaching from what I was feeling in my body. Not only was I more 'in my head' than 'in my body', but I knew that my left brain was taking over, the side which needs rules, defined structures and works in a very linear way. My right brain, with its creativity and problem-solving capacity, along with the wisdom of my body, was effectively lost to me, a shift that resulted in old habits resurfacing. I shut down, withdrew and retreated from the world.

The fact that these behaviours returned also revealed that despite what I thought, I'd never learnt how to navigate conflict in a healthy way. On the contrary, I would still run from the slightest hint of it. Conflict scared me and was a stark reminder of the volatile atmosphere in which I had grown up. I didn't know how to have difficult conversations, ask assertively but respectfully for my needs to be met, and explore ways to find a healthy compromise. Though I did my best (and in some way, I felt I was being assertive and respectful), it became obvious it wasn't working.

I think, at the time, I was coming from a place of fear and victimhood, which explained why I wasn't getting anywhere. If, instead, I'd been able to come from a place of knowing my worth (as opposed to doubting my place and merits as a stepmother) and feeling free to be both loving and compassionate towards myself, my husband and our relationship, then things would have looked a little different. I would, I believe, have avoided the inevitable side-effect of this situation, which was an increase in my anxiety and the desire to start self-harming as a way to manage my feelings (which is never a healthy strategy).

My life felt unpredictable and uncertain, and as though everything was out of my control. I felt unsupported, alone, powerless, with no one caring enough to listen. I was also angry and ashamed that my marriage was falling apart for the second time, and I didn't seem able to save it. I was right back to being the child who had felt ugly and unworthy.

It was within the depths of this dark, miserable place that I went to the doctor. I was given medication and again referred for counselling, but once more, I found these had little to no effect. The medication and counselling weren't helping me to reframe my perception; in fact, it felt as if they were reinforcing it through the need for me to revisit old wounds. Equally, they weren't giving me back any sense of autonomy, and I found myself even more dependent and helpless than ever.

It was during this second experience of counselling and medication that I had one of the most profound understandings of my life. I realised that my current perspective of feeling powerless, worthless and sorry for myself was not serving me at all, and, in the same way as I had done during my illnesses, I searched for a better way of looking at my situation. Again, I didn't know what I was looking for, but I wanted to feel more grounded, centred, autonomous and happy, and I knew that if I continued on my existing path, I would become ill.

My friends and family tried to support me, but what we don't often understand is that this can sometimes hold us back. Sympathy, however well-intended, can prevent us from moving forward. Having our feelings validated feels affirming, but if it doesn't then help us to move forward and make supportive changes, it can actually stop us from progressing. If our position and feelings (of pain) are reinforced, then this can actually increase our sense of powerlessness, even to the point where we see ourselves as victims of our own situation.

But – and this is where things really began to change - I didn't want to feel that way. I'd had enough of being powerless, so instead, I started to be really honest with myself. I knew, for example, that my loved ones were only hearing one side of the story – my side – but I wasn't the only one in the situation with a valid perspective. My husband and stepson, my work colleagues, my family - they all had a perspective, too. Where was the space for them to be heard and their opinions considered?

Though I could only effect change in myself, I knew that mutual understanding and acceptance with everyone in my life was what I wanted. I felt strongly that it was important to consider other people's perspectives, too, and perhaps, if I did this, I would discover a way to find balance and healing for myself.

I started out on a quest to find something that would shift things within me to a better place. I don't know if I really believed I could achieve change, but I was kind of out of options, and so, with the energy and determination of the desperate, I set off.

It was at this point that I returned to the inner core of Love from Walsch's Conversations with God. Could I find it, and if so, could I live in that place? Would it be the answer to the hurts of my past and the dis-ease that they had created? Could I do this without the need for medication or painful, shame-inducing sessions of therapy?

I knew little at this point other than I wanted to take back control of my life and feel grounded, balanced, uplifted and supported. I wanted to understand myself in a way that allowed me to gain a sense of agency and be my best Self. This, I believed, would lead me to the happiness I longed for whilst also allowing space for others' thoughts and opinions. In short, I was looking for physical, mental, emotional and spiritual healing and wellbeing.

So, what did I find?

Well, having started with few expectations, I ended up finding a rich and abundant treasure trove, which is what I'll be sharing with you over the next few chapters. The beauty of this treasure is that it's available to everyone, though it may take a bit of digging to reach. Sometimes, during this process – which I often liken to spring cleaning - things may seem messier before they improve, but at each step along the way, you will develop a new understanding, a deeper self-compassion, and the internal healing that is unique to you.

Chapter Summary

We learned:

- The messy, tangled, overgrown roots from which my journey started.
- How navigating from this spot can make it tricky to figure out the path to meaningful changes and picture a brighter future.
- As we continue through the book, I hope you'll start to notice that even small tweaks and additions to your daily routine can make a significant difference. These subtle changes can lead to positive, step-by-step shifts, bringing you closer to your wellbeing goals.

~ Two ~
Work With What You've Got
The Journey Towards W·I·L·D®

Inside Chapter Two

Within Chapter 2, we will be exploring some of the concepts that underpin my work, healing and journey. We look in more depth at the following:

- *the foundation of W·I·L·D®.*

- *how our perception impacts on our experience.*

- *the importance of becoming grounded and centred in order to support ourselves on our wellbeing journey.*

There will be several examples to illustrate how you might approach this process.

~ ~ ~ ~ ~

So, there I was, embarking on this journey with only the most general sense of where I wanted to get to and with no directions, map or compass to guide me. I felt inadequately prepared and had no idea how long it would take to get to my destination, but the thing I had in my favour was that I knew I was starting with an open mind. I also had no expectations and intended to work with what I had rather than focusing – as I was previously – on all the things that I wanted but didn't have. That route had only brought misery and frustration, so it was time to try a different way.

Having read *'Conversations with God'* by Neale Donald Walsch,

I 'somehow' came across a nine-month online programme called Evolutionary Enlightenment, led by Craig Hamilton, which was based on the book of the same name written by Andrew Cohen. I think of this as being one of those wonderful 'co-incidences' (i.e., things that happen together – 'co-incide' - with beautiful synchronicity as a gift from the Universe). It was just one example of many in my life which have illustrated the truth of the saying:

'When the student is ready, the teacher will appear'

I decided to enrol on this programme and learnt so much during the nine months, which helped to broaden my perspective and understanding exponentially. One example centred around studying the two concepts of the **Relative Self** and the **Absolute Self**.

The **Relative Self** is the part of us that exists here and now, while the **Absolute Self** is the part of us that exists outside of time and space. This Absolute Self is the part of us that has never been and, in fact, can never be broken.

Absolute Self can be understood along these lines: Einstein said that 'Energy cannot be created or destroyed; it can only be changed from one form to another.'

Everything is made of energy, including us. If we are to believe Einstein and our 'energy can only be changed from one form to another', there is a part of us that is arguably eternal. It can never be destroyed. It can never die. It just changes form or state. If we believe this, then we can see that there is a part of us that exists outside of time and space. This is how I understand the Absolute Self.

Also, I see the creative force of Life - the Universe, Source, God, or whatever name you give to the wonder of all that we see around us - as being like a vast ocean, with each of us as a drop within that ocean. Each of us is a part of the Creative Energy of Life that is constantly learning, growing and evolving, adding our own unique flavour to the world by our presence here.

These observations lead me to believe that we have (at least) two layers of being – our physical presence in the world and our spiritual energy (or essence) that is part of the greater Life Energy. Our spiritual energy is indestructible, and it can never be broken, whereas our physical self lives in a 'relative' world where we experience light and dark, hot and cold, joy and sorrow, and so on. Our Absolute Self just is – it is constant and unchanging.

This is an important point, and understanding Relative Self vs Absolute Self can be difficult, but it may help to think of it in terms of experiences and contrasts. For example, we need to know darkness in order to know light, sorrow to appreciate joy, and so on, all of which happen in the physical world, yet there is a part of us that forms the 'bigger picture'. This is the part which allows us to make choices that are less clouded by the intensity of the moment by tuning into our 'absolute' or 'bigger picture' self. Being the more objective 'observer' of the situation if you like. This, for me, is the difference between our Physical and Absolute Selves. I saw (and still do see) this concept as being the same as Walsch's, 'Who I Really Am', for it is the part of us that is 'of the Divine'[1].

Going back to the Evolutionary Enlightenment course, we were encouraged to regularly view things from the perspective of our Absolute Self or, another version, from the perspective of our Deathbed-self. Whilst this may sound rather morbid, the concept is more about looking back over life to see which bits really mattered when viewed in our final days. From there, from our deathbed, our day-to-day struggles and disagreements will often fade into insignificance, raising the question of why we put so much of our daily energy and focus into things which eventually will not matter to us. (If this idea is of interest to you, you might like to read *The Top Five Regrets of the Dying: A Life Transformed by the Dearly Departing*' by Bronnie Ware).

Once I understood the concept, viewing things from this perspective

---

1   By 'Divine' I simply mean that creative Life Energy. You might think of it as God, Universe, Source, or some other name, but essentially it is whatever you associate with 'spiritual'. For me this is separate from 'religion' and is more a question of 'belief' or 'faith'. I came across a beautiful quote some years ago that summed this up for me: 'A spiritual practice is anything that makes you feel more beautiful inside you.' – Sri Avinash Do.

was liberating. It offered me a greater sense of simplicity and proportion, which enabled clarity of what was truly important and, thus, where I needed to focus my energy and attention. I found that the other 'unnecessary' details would then just fall away – even if only temporarily – but it was enough to help me feel more centred. Since then, I've been a great lover of simplicity in all things.

To give an example of how the Deathbed-self concept works (for me) - I was planning a trip to Ireland to visit family. Work was busy, with several deadlines and events coming up, and I was feeling a little anxious about leaving Dax and Rika (my horses) in the care of my 'non-horsey' husband. For the first time ever, Mum would be unable to pick me up from the airport, so I started thinking about hiring a car, something I'd never done before. This, coupled with my concerns about leaving the horses, meant that my brain was juggling several elements, and I was fast approaching overwhelm. Turning to the deathbed-self concept, I asked myself the following questions:

- am I worrying about things that are outside of my control?
- am I taking on things that aren't my responsibility?
- can I divide the situation into smaller 'chunks' and deal with each one separately?
- can I ask for/accept help from other people?

And that's when the whole idea began to make sense. I discovered that exploring the answers to these questions helped me find ways to reduce my stress and make everything feel much more manageable, thus giving me a greater sense of breathing space, time and agency (control) in the situation. The end result was that I was able to relax and enjoy the time with my family rather than worrying about all the things which I could do nothing about.

From my studies and other reading that I did around this time (including Eckhart Tolle's excellent book, 'The Power of Now'), I began to understand that, in themselves, things which had happened in my life weren't 'good' or 'bad' – they just were. It was me who assigned meaning to them.

I was the one who labelled them 'good' or 'bad', 'wanted' or 'unwanted', and as such, I was creating the suffering I was experiencing.

To illustrate, I'd like to share a couple of things:

Fact:

Life will always throw us curveballs. It can get messy, and it can be uncomfortable, but this is just how it is. However, if we get upset by these curveballs and start to attach negative feelings to the resulting messiness and discomfort, these 'facts of life' will turn into suffering. Through my learnings, I began to understand that pain was the experience, whereas suffering was my interpretation of it, i.e., it's the meaning that I – and you - put onto our pain. When we assign 'meaning' to something, rather than taking it as a simple fact over which there is no control, this can cause us to feel bad about feeling bad, which doubles our discomfort. Additionally, it can lead us to look for something or someone to blame.

I recognised that this was exactly what I had been doing.

"Pain is inevitable. Suffering is optional."

(Haruki Murakami, Japanese writer and translator.)

I mentioned earlier that Abraham-Hicks teaches, *'a belief is only a thought I keep thinking'*, which I liken to a circle, known as the Thought-Belief Cycle:

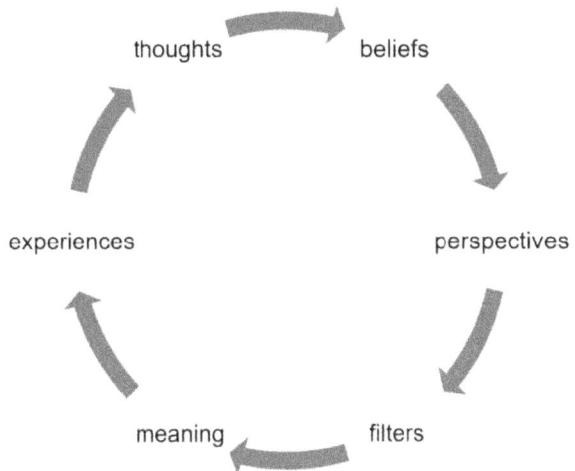

thoughts → beliefs → perspectives → filters → meaning → experiences → thoughts

This is how it works:

What we **think** creates our **beliefs**, which determine our **perspective**, which in turn constructs the **filters**, or lenses, through which we see the world. This determines the **meaning** that we put on what happens to us, which we then record as our **experiences**. These then influence the thoughts we have about the world in which we live and the people we encounter, which then determines what we **think** … and so the cycle repeats endlessly. Unless that is, we consciously decide to interrupt the cycle and change it in some way. Interrupting this cycle is something we will be exploring later in this book.

I've also realised that our thoughts aren't actually where this circle 'begins'. The thing that comes first is a feeling. Think of it like this:

Our bodies are always the first part of us to respond to our environment. The sensations and emotions we feel aren't 'right' or 'wrong', 'good' or 'bad', they just are. These feelings are our body's way of communicating with us, letting us know whether what's going on in our environment feels safe or not.

As human beings, we then go on to attach meaning to these sensations and to any external events which activated them. There's nothing wrong with this, but it's helpful to remember that when we experience the disconnect of trauma (when we're left feeling deep shame and don't think we can talk to anyone about what's happened, or we've dissociated[2] because we feel totally overwhelmed), our brains become wired into a sense of lack of safety, and we become hypervigilant and fearful. This can result in us attaching meanings to the sensations or emotions which are negatively biased, and we can then come to see these as 'truth' when, in fact, they may only exist in our head.

For example, I mentioned in the last chapter that I found the shifting friendships of the school playground difficult to navigate. This was due to my experiences when I was very small and I'd come to believe that

2 Dissociation is a concept that has been developed over time and concerns a wide array of experiences, ranging from a mild emotional detachment from the immediate surroundings to a more severe disconnection from physical and emotional experiences - Wikipedia

I wasn't good enough. When someone I'd thought of as 'my friend' went off to play with someone else, I interpreted this as meaning they had come to see my flaws, so they had rejected me to find a better friend. This left me feeling deeply hurt and more worthless than ever, and also more watchful for any possible signs that I might be rejected again. As a result, I became more of a loner and was very slow to trust and build friendships. In reality, my friend who had decided to play with someone else wasn't thinking any of these things – especially at that age when we are far from a level of emotional maturity to even formulate these thoughts – yet by attaching negative thoughts to the situation I exacerbated the resulting feelings which led to a more difficult time at school.

As you can no doubt see, all too easily this becomes a downward spiral of anxiety that is hard to break out of without support. This is because when we are in such a spiral, we can be too close to the problem, and become so caught up in the intensity of the emotions that we are unable to retain the necessary level of clarity. If we reach this point and decide to work with a practitioner, it is imperative to find one with whom we feel safe and who allows us to work through things in a gentle and compassionate way. Getting to the root of the issue always involves exploring deep feelings – feelings we might have worked hard to avoid for a long time – and this can be painful, messy and even scary, but when we know that we are safely held (by the support of a trained professional), it becomes possible to do the necessary exploration and achieve deep and lasting healing. My early experience of counselling was not as supportive as I needed, which is why, on reflection, I gained little in respect of healing from it.

I have to admit it took me a long time to understand that I could choose my perspective; that, if I find my experience uncomfortable, I can change my thoughts about it or alter the meaning I give to it, which will result in a different feeling. This realisation has been a step-by-step, layer-by-layer process, and there are still challenges which catch me out from time to time.

Sometimes it can be difficult to fit our challenges/feelings/emotions/experiences into the framework of the **Thought-Belief cycle**, but as a rule of thumb, I always remember that we struggle more when we are close to those challenges – when they 'push our buttons' in some way.

I use the Thought-Belief cycle extensively for myself and in my work, so when it happens that I cannot make whatever I am experiencing 'fit', then I try to laugh with myself about how I have reacted before getting curious about what further wisdom this reaction might have to share with me.

At this point, you may be wondering how this works, how you fit your challenge or situation into the cycle in order to change your perspective and how you, too, can navigate the process. As an illustration, for me, it works like this:

1. I start by noticing how I'm feeling. When we tune in to notice our physical and emotional sensations, they can give us so much valuable information. Later in the book, I share a Body Scan exercise, which is an excellent tool for doing this, but for now, simply try listening to your body. The more you do, the more you can build up an understanding of how you feel at each emotional stage – how you feel when you're happy and things are going well and how you notice that you are not in that place.

2. If you notice a feeling of discomfort, this is an opportunity to get curious and compassionately explore what you are thinking and what beliefs you're holding about the situation.

3. Take a moment to sit with each thought/belief. If it leaves you feeling 'less' in some way, for example, less happy, worthy, positive or good about yourself, then explore how you could reframe it to being something that feels even a little better. You might find the Emotion Scale opposite helpful here.

4. From here, every time you notice yourself thinking the old thought, practice replacing it with the new one. (The exercise in Appendix 4 can be very helpful here.)

5. It's important to remember to stay curious and compassionate. We can often beat ourselves up if we find it difficult to shift old patterns but remember that it took time to create those old thoughts and beliefs, and it will take time to embed new ones. In fact, it takes at least 21 days to build a new habit.

> **TIP**: Try to focus on the new habit you're creating rather than fighting to change the old one. You'll be able to see the effects of this exercise by how you feel and by how your reactions to situations begin to shift. This might be subtle at first, but over time, if you look back, you'll be able to see the change. Or, you might even find that others comment on it, saying that you're calmer, happier or more relaxed, for example. It's about keeping an open mind rather than having any expectation to agree or disagree with a particular set of beliefs.

THE EMOTION SCALE

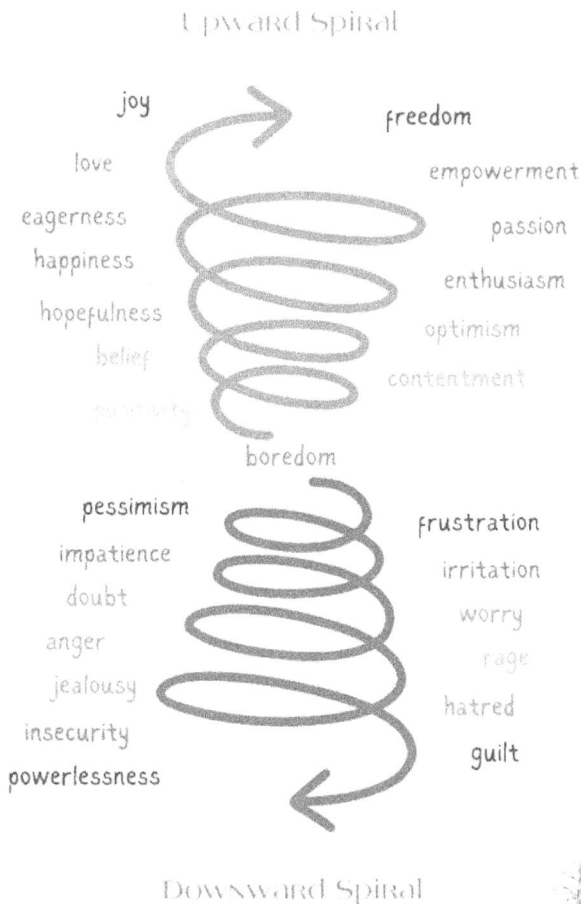

Upward Spiral

joy

freedom

love

empowerment

eagerness

passion

happiness

enthusiasm

hopefulness

optimism

belief

contentment

boredom

pessimism

frustration

impatience

irritation

doubt

worry

anger

rage

jealousy

hatred

insecurity

guilt

powerlessness

Downward Spiral

Part of my healing journey involved going to see an amazing doctor – Dr Magee - in Belfast. He was trained in mainstream medicine but also brought other approaches into his practice, and it was he who first introduced me to *energy* as something that I could feel. Prior to this, I'd thought of energy as something that powered batteries or electric circuits - it's what flows when we flick a switch, and the light comes on, right? Or how we heat our homes and power our fridges and televisions?

But this doctor gave me a new understanding. He demonstrated that energy is an amazing force we can all feel in our bodies. He took time with me, listening and explaining, and I left his clinic buzzing with questions: What did it mean? What was this force of energy? How could I feel it, and what might it mean for me and the possibility of long-term healing?

I wanted to know more so I began my study of Reiki[3] in the quest for answers. Not only did I end up becoming qualified in Reiki to Practitioner level, but it had another unforeseen result. Reiki reconnected me with animals.

I mentioned earlier that when I was growing up, I found it difficult to make friends and found it hard to trust people and be open enough to connect with them. With animals though, I felt completely safe. They didn't ask anything of me, and they didn't judge – they just accepted me for who I was.

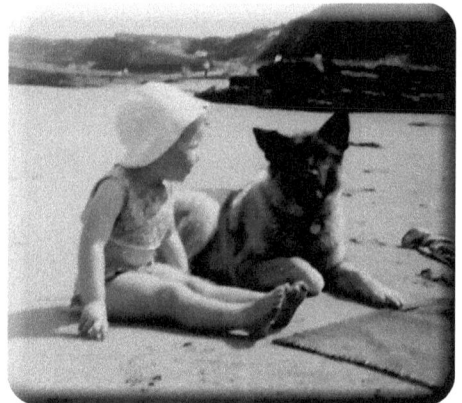

I grew up with the most wonderful dog, Mitzi, who was my equivalent of Nana from Peter Pan.

After she died, we got a cat, Topaz, and later another dog, Tam. Friends

---

3   *"Reiki is a Japanese technique for stress reduction and relaxation that also promotes healing. It is administered by "laying on hands" and is based on the idea that an unseen "life force energy" flows through us and is what causes us to be alive. If one's "life force energy" is low, then we are more likely to get sick or feel stress, and if it is high, we are more capable of being happy and healthy." Source: www.reiki.org*

and family had dogs, too, plus Mum knew people with horses and ponies, and when I was old enough, she paid for me to have weekly riding lessons. All of these animals became my playmates and 'safe space', often replacing the human company I found so hard to come by.

When I went away to university, I lost touch with this part of myself and became convinced that it didn't matter, but when Reiki reopened this powerful connection, I realised I was mistaken and that I needed animals to be a part of my life. Eventually, they also became part of my search for greater wellbeing.

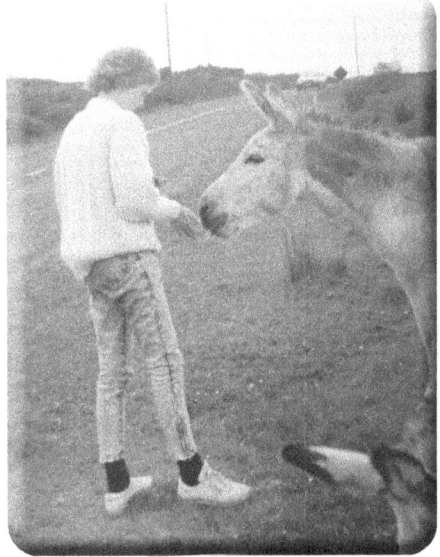

In January 2011, the world aligned once more when I came across an animal communication workshop that was taking place near Guildford. This was around the time of Mum's 70th birthday, and knowing that this would interest her, I asked if she'd like to come over from Ireland, spend a couple of nights in a B&B and attend this course with me. She accepted, and that weekend, I met Julie Lines (now Jules Chabeaux), who would go on to become a wonderful, supportive and inspirational friend.

The workshop itself was held on a rare breed farm where we connected with pigs, turkeys, ferrets, horses and a gorgeous spaniel who insisted on sitting on my lap for the whole of his session! I was in heaven. Jules and I began talking about my studies in Reiki and the possibility of using this with animals, and from this, she recommended I study energy healing with The Healing Trust (NFSH). Not only would I learn so much, but it would also provide me with a recognised qualification acknowledged by vets, meaning I could work with animals as part of my healing practice. I was sold! - and commenced a fabulous course in Bristol, which included tons of new information that I hadn't learnt through my Reiki studies.

During this course, we studied anatomy and physiology as well as working with the energy of colours, which is fascinating.

My book editor, for example, asked what the energy interpretation was for the colour green, in particular lime green (her favourite colour), and I was able to provide her with this response based on the learnings from The Healing Trust qualification.

Green is the colour of nature and healing (it boosts the immune system)—it's why medics often use this colour—uniforms, pharmacy signs, etc. It also relates to forward movement and growth—think of traffic lights and plants. Also, green relates to self-esteem/self-respect, and it can help us narrow down our focus. Lime green contains a lot of yellow, which is a colour of opening, expansion, freedom, and looking to the future.

See? Fascinating.

After completing the course in Bristol, I returned for a further Animal Communication weekend with Jules, which focused solely on horses, these being the animals to which I felt most deeply drawn.

Following this, my tutor with The Healing Trust pointed me in the direction of Liz Whiter from the Healing Animals Organisation, suggesting this would be a great place to start if I wanted to work professionally with horses—which I did.

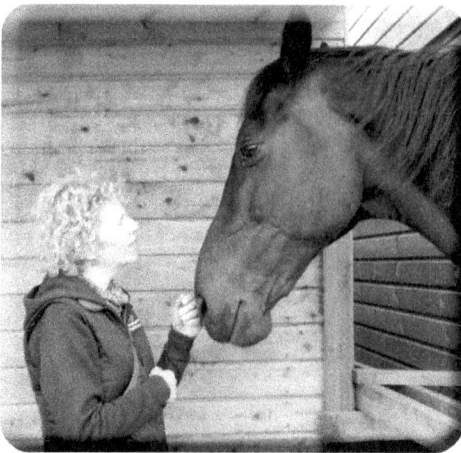

I ended up doing the HAO diploma in small animal healing, followed by a specialist course in equines with further training in equine massage and a taster day on acupressure. I felt so blessed to be soaking up this fabulous learning, which now feeds into the work I do, both with people, horses and other animals. (If you'd like to know more about this, read my article on *Giving Wellbeing Some Horse Power* - see Resources list at the end of the book for the link.)

Two significant further shifts came while I was working with a therapist—Linda Burke—in Enniskillen, Northern Ireland. The first of these happened when she referred me to a colleague of hers who was a practitioner of 'MetaHealth'. His name was Richard Flook, and he'd written a great book explaining this 'MetaHealth' approach titled '*Why Am I Sick*'.

Following Linda's introduction, Richard sent me to have a CT scan of my brain, which was analysed in a very particular way to reveal where I was holding traumas from my earlier life that still impacted me. I was also asked to put together my personal timeline, and this, along with the CT results, allowed Richard to compile a report for me on what was happening in my body and why. Then, he explained, I would be able to understand and begin to address any changes necessary.

The report blew me away! For the first time in my life, I felt truly seen and understood on a profound internal level by another person, even though he had only met me once. Somehow, from the scan and timeline, he'd been able to identify the emotional things (happenings/events) that I'd never talked about—or even fully recognised myself. This enabled me to witness my pain and really honour and appreciate this for the first time.

Before this, I was a classic minimiser. I'd think and say things like: 'Other people have been through much worse' or 'That's all in the past', but for my body, what I had experienced obviously had a significant impact and was still present - and visible - in my brain.

The second shift was when, during one of our sessions, Linda asked me:

"What do you like to do? Where is your happy place?"

At that point, I was in such a low place that part of me just wanted to shout, "Nothing!".

But from somewhere deep inside of me, another voice spoke:

"Nature", it said.

I still don't really know where this came from; it wasn't as if I spent much time outdoors at that point, and if the weather was grey or wet, I would positively avoid it. Perhaps my inner child remembered walks, picnics, games and time spent with dogs and horses and longed for the sense of safety, belonging and space that they'd once given me. Whatever it was, the therapist and I ran with it and explored how I might bring more 'Nature' into my life, assigning me the task of turning our garden, a square of very damp grass and moss, into a wildlife garden.

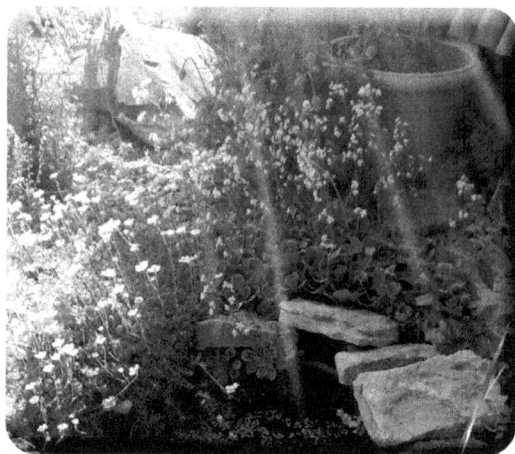

'Yeah, right!' I thought. 'My husband's not going to go for this!' (He'd previously told me to leave this square as it was because he and his son used it for playing football!)

Astonishingly, when I broached the subject, I was to be proved wrong (possibly helped by the fact that his son was getting too big to play football in that space – which was confirmed not long afterwards by a broken kitchen window). Football was thus moved to the green space on the other side of our hedge, and I was given free rein in the garden.

Over the next couple of years, I transformed that very damp square of green into a wildlife garden complete with trellis, herbs and a pond. It was such wonderful therapy and taught me so much about what makes me happy. I will always be grateful to Linda for this suggestion.

Shortly thereafter, I realised that this therapy and my new practice of self-care were having a dramatic effect. The IBS, migraines, and eczema, which used to flare up quite regularly, slowly faded away. As I began listening to my body with increased awareness, I made tweaks to my lifestyle that felt right for me. Two significant changes I made were becoming a vegan and learning the importance of taking time for myself. I knew I was feeling the best I had in years.

> **Author Note**: *I'd like to say here that this is very much a personal journey and is about finding out what's right for you. Becoming a vegan, for example, works for me, but it's not the right choice for everyone. If you do change your diet, it's important to make sure that whatever you choose to eat, your nutritional intake is well-balanced and provides everything your body needs.*

I was so grateful for all I had learnt and for everyone who supported my education and growth that it became an easy decision to set up *Equenergy* in 2013 to pass these teachings and knowledge on to others. *Equenergy* is a play on words, fusing equilibrium (balance) and energy. When we learn how to bring our energies back into balance, it supports our healing and brings greater wellbeing.

The business has changed a lot since then (including the name, it's now W•I•L•D® Wellbeing), but the creation of Equenergy was the start of me exploring what I could share from my own journey that would be of value to others who found themselves where I had been - in that dark, lonely, unhappy place where everything feels hope-less and help-less.

As my practice grew, I knew that I loved using energy work and Reiki, but I also wanted to add further tools that I could use to support people and help them develop their own self-care 'toolkit'. This desire led me to the *Emotional Freedom Technique* (EFT, also known as 'tapping') and *Matrix Reimprinting* (MR). Both of these techniques use the same meridian lines as traditional Chinese acupuncture but without the need for needles. They are highly effective therapies which can be used for a wide range of issues such as allergies, phobias, pain and anxiety - without side effects.

As a vegan and lover of animals and Nature, as well as being passionate about wellbeing, I was also on the lookout for healthier products to use (both on ourselves and in our homes). Browsing social media, I happened upon a tweet about Arbonne, a network marketing company selling cosmetics, toiletries and health supplements, so I contacted Liz, the author of the tweet, and we arranged to meet. After learning more about the company's products and ethos, I decided to join, and along the way, Liz and I became friends.

Sometime later, Liz told me that a fantastic health and wellness trainer from London would be running a workshop at her house. She needed to get enough people together for it to be viable and wondered if I'd be interested in coming along. The topic of the workshop was MetaHealth! Remembering the impact of my previous experience with MetaHealth (having the CT scan and reading the subsequent report), of course, I was interested. I signed up and proceeded to go through the most eye-opening, life-changing training I've ever experienced. That workshop pulled together (and made sense of) my whole journey up to that point. (MetaHealth has now evolved further, thanks to the trainer I studied with - Penny Croal of Change Ahead - who has called her branch of this practice *Meta Consciousness®*.)

Throughout this journey, from stress and poor health to healing and qualifying as a wellbeing practitioner, I constantly learnt, changed and grew. I went from being in a space that felt restricted, dark and alone to somewhere where I felt connected, lighter and more expansive. I recognised that Nature was so much a part of where I was, and I longed to immerse myself further in her healing energy. Moreover, I wanted to create a space to share this with others.

It seemed only natural to bring animals into my life. Firstly, a fabulous feline, Kali, who was an incredible teacher. In typical cat fashion, she was a wonderful role model for being your true self and doing what's right for you, no matter what anyone else thinks. I then took on a rescue horse, Dakota (Dax), who I initially kept in a livery yard about three miles away; however, I knew I wanted him to be with us on our own land, so my husband and I started looking for a new home. After much searching, we found the beautiful place we are in now, situated in glorious rural Wales, ten minutes outside of Abergavenny and just inside the fabulous Brecon Beacons National Park. With the addition of Rika, my second horse, this was a dream come true. Not only did I get everything I needed for my own wellbeing – Nature and animals being the most important – but I can also share this magical and healing space with the people and animals who come to me.

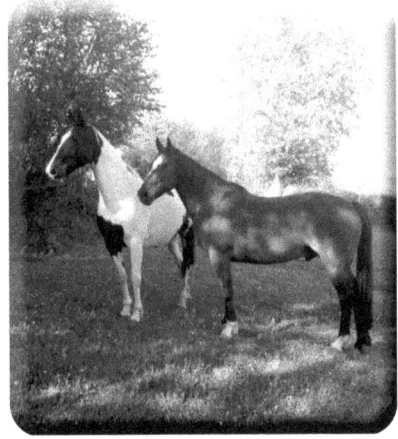

And so, you are pretty much up to date. The point we have reached is where Equenergy: W·I·L·D® Wellbeing was born. Without further ado, therefore, we will start digging into the nuts and bolts of this practice.

(Remember, the journey you are embarking on is yours. Feel free to take from my story only the things that resonate with you and discard the rest. You can also 'adopt and adapt' any elements. The important thing is to enjoy the ride.)

Let's take a Walk on the W·I·L·D® side!

Chapter Summary

We looked at:

- The impact of our perception on our experience.
- The *Thought–Belief Cycle* and *The Emotion Scale* help us build towards emotional self-awareness. Think of this as a sturdy foundation to propel you forward, something you can always revisit to reground and centre yourself. Feel free to dive deeper into these concepts as you progress along your journey.

~ Three ~
What is W·I·L·D®?

Inside Chapter Three

In this chapter, I explore a fundamental aspect: cultivating a Sense of Safety – not just physically but emotionally and psychologically. Without this foundation, we will not be able to reach our fullest potential.

~ ~ ~ ~ ~

"What is this 'W·I·L·D®'?" I hear you ask.

It's actually really simple. It's the acronym I created for all the things Mother Nature has taught me about healing and wellbeing. It's not a set of steps exactly, simply because I don't believe in a 'one-size-fits-all' approach. We are all unique individuals with our own particular needs and preferences, so W·I·L·D® is more a way of 'being' that brings you back to your centre. It guides you towards feeling more comfortable within your own skin and becoming the person you were born to be. Your personal healing is supported by this process, which means greater wellbeing and joy in your life going forward.

I think we often spend too much time in our own headspace trying to analyse, rationalise and work things out logically, which isn't wrong - there's most definitely a valid place for it – however, I personally feel it's important to spend more time on things which help us to bring more BE-ing into our lives.

But what does BE-ing mean?

For me, it's about stepping into that earlier concept from Neale Donald

Walsch – the idea of *'Who I Really Am'* – and exploring how we can live more from that place. It's about embracing our True Nature and giving ourselves permission to BE this and to celebrate all of who we are – the weirdness, the messiness and the wonder of every aspect of our being.

I spoke earlier about Gabor Maté whose work has had a huge impact on me. One concept he references is our True Nature and observes that discomfort comes when we are not aligned with this. A bit like the 'lane assist' function in some cars, for example. If your car has this facility, an alarm will sound if you start to veer out of your lane. This is because its function is to alert the driver to potential danger in case they've fallen asleep at the wheel or their attention was elsewhere, for example.

Discomfort (whether that be physical, emotional, psychological, or social) is the same; it is an alert signal that lets us know we are 'drifting out of our lane'.

If we continue to 'drift out of our lane', we are potentially wearing a mask, i.e., not BE-ing ourselves, and can thus be putting others' needs before our own, which usually doesn't serve us. My own personal belief is that we're each here to bring something unique to the world, that we have our own particular light to shine, yet if we're not being faithful to Who We Really Are, if we've drifted away from our *True Nature* (out of our lane), we can find it hard to be our Unique Self. And not being our *Unique Self* is where it begins to hurt because this is where we can start to feel 'off' and unfulfilled like something inside of us is longing to get out and express itself. One of the main reasons I developed W·I·L·D® is to enable us all to find our Unique Self, which is a thread you will see and follow throughout the next chapters.

Let's start, though, by looking at what might take us out of our lane and away from our Unique Self and True Nature.

As infants, we all have two basic needs: *Attachment* and *Authenticity* (The Myth of Normal, pp105-109). At this young age, we're not able to change our personal situation, so if we ever feel that being Authentic (true to what we want/need) threatens our Attachment - i.e., if we feel that by expressing our personal needs, fears or emotions, we will lose connection with our caregiver - then we will sacrifice our Authenticity in order to maintain the Attachment. Why? Because at that young age, we do not have the tools to survive on our own, thus this abandonment of authenticity as an infant is not a conscious choice. It is survival.

As a simple example, a two-year-old may be frustrated that she is unable to ask for what she wants in words, so she stamps her foot and begins to cry loudly. If her parent berates her, telling her that such behaviour is unacceptable and that 'nice girls' don't show their temper in such a way, the child might end up suppressing her feelings (of frustration in this case) in order to maintain a connection with her parent. At the age of two, she hasn't yet learnt how to navigate her feelings healthily or to understand them and appreciate the information they offer. Instead, she's being taught that to keep the peace and her caregiver happy, she needs to push down those feelings. This can lead to the child (subconsciously) suppressing her emotions because expressing them could trigger the loss of a safe connection with her parent/caregiver. In this way, she is disconnecting from her True Nature. Whilst this is a natural strategy for the child to develop in such a situation - given the limited tools she has at her disposal - it isn't a healthy one. You can see from this example how the young child has traded her authenticity for attachment without conscious knowledge, which can potentially create a default behaviour of ignoring her True Nature throughout life.

It is my belief that personal healing comes from finding ways to reconnect with our True Nature and, through this, with our communities and the World in which we live. This healing can then extend beyond us as we start to get a clear and supportive understanding of our unique sense of Self, Place, and Belonging.

And this unique sense of Self, Place and Belonging is what W·I·L·D® offers us.

Our sense of Self, Place and Belonging can, like Nature herself, be challenging to tie down. It can feel 'messy' and 'untamed' at times, but ultimately, if you embrace their W·I·L·D®ness, you'll see these don't need to be static things. It's okay for them to be fluid and flexible and to go through times of uncertainty and readjustment. Then, you will realise what it is to be exquisitely, magnificently, magically, and gloriously beautiful.

I referenced 'safety' at the beginning of this chapter, and before we dive in and explore W·I·L·D® in greater depth, it's important to spend a few moments focusing on what I mean by 'safety' and why it is so crucial. Although you might be tempted to skip past this part so that you can get into the nitty gritty of W·I·L·D®, I would encourage you not to. Your safety, in all its forms, is key both in your progression through W·I·L·D® but also in ensuring you can achieve the most beneficial outcome.

For the purposes of this book and my work, there are three key aspects to safety: physical safety, emotional safety and psychological safety – which will become apparent as we go through this next section. First though, let's look at what 'safety' means.

Safety First

The Oxford English Dictionary defines safety as:

"The state of being protected from or guarded against hurt or injury; freedom from danger."

In the context of this book, I use the term 'safety' to refer to the state of 'feeling safe', that is:

- at ease, comfortable and 'at home' within your own body and the spaces you inhabit and;
- freedom from any sense of threat, worry, danger or anxiety of a physical, emotional or psychological nature.

If you've experienced the kind of deep disconnection that I talked about in Chapter 1, if you've felt isolated, alone or anxious, or if you've experienced imposter syndrome or shame, please pay particular attention to this section.

Similarly, if you experienced Childhood Emotional Neglect (CEN), if you have a moderate to high 'ACE' score (ACE stands for Adverse Childhood Experiences)[1], or if you've been diagnosed with AD(H) D, PTSD, ASD, BPD or bipolar disorder, then this part is also important for you.

Even if you don't believe you fall into either of these camps, try to remember that we all use words in different ways and attach different meanings or associations to them. One person's 'anxious' might be another person's 'nervous' or even 'excited', so it can be useful to focus on the impact our feelings have on us.

Understanding Our Reactions

Do you find yourself reacting (to perceived threats) from a deeply ingrained conditioned behaviour, or are you able to consider your response to a given situation and consciously choose what you say or do? It's worth taking a moment to really consider this. Perhaps imagine yourself in different situations, think about what would cause you to feel threatened (i.e. not safe) and consider how you would react.

If you find you are repeating unconscious patterns of behaviour (especially those which are not serving you) then this in itself can be an indication of holding onto past events which are still impacting you today – and this is often the cause of our issues.

In her book *Braving The Wilderness*, Brené Brown talks about having a 'strong back, a soft front and a wild heart' (Chapter 7). She describes how, when we feel threatened, we can have a default reaction of 'armouring up' (pg. 153-4). Other variations might be to 'puff up' or 'shrink'. Given that I see Nature and animals as such great teachers, I often use visuals to help me understand reactions and behaviours. A simple way to think of this is as follows:

- I visualise an inflated puffer fish to better relate to the 'puffing up' behaviour.

---

1 *If you'd like to do a test to discover your ACE score, there are various options available on the internet, such as this one from Harvard University: https://developingchild.harvard.edu/media-coverage/take-the-ace-quiz-and-learn-what-it-does-and-doesnt-mean/)*

- I visualise a crab with its claws raised in defence for 'armouring up'.
- I visualise a tortoise pulling back into its shell for 'shrinking'.

If you imagine your reaction in these terms, it can be much easier to work out which is your default or 'go-to' reaction when you feel threatened.

When I attributed visuals (animals) to these phrases, I was able to figure out that my preferred and default go-to reaction when threatened was to 'shrink'. If, however, that didn't feel like an option, then I would 'puff up' to try and deter any perceived threat, and if that wasn't enough, then I might, as a last resort, 'armour up'.

Using this visual imagery helps me to understand my reactions more clearly, and I still use it today. It really helps me to simplify my behaviours by aligning them with the visceral habits of animals because, essentially, we as humans have the same.

Even knowing this, I still found that none of the strategies I was using, worked.

- 'Shrinking' meant that I didn't get to express what I was feeling or what I wanted.
- 'Armouring up' was exhausting and limiting because it didn't allow me to learn or grow.
- 'Puffing up' was tiring and left me with feelings of Imposter Syndrome, fearing that someone would discover the truth about me.

Ultimately, I was concerned that those shameful things we hope no one will ever discover about us - such as our innermost fears, weaknesses or secret beliefs, likes and dislikes, which might mark us as different from our peers - would be revealed or challenged.

So, what can you do if you recognise yourself using these or similar behaviours and find them equally as unhelpful as I did? How can you shift from these unconscious behaviours towards something which will enable you to step into healthier, more conscious responses that allow you to grow and heal?

I mentioned earlier that there are three aspects of safety: *physical*, *emotional* and *psychological*, and it was whilst I was researching these that I began to uncover just how important an appreciation of our 'sense of safety' is and how I believe this forms a basis for our subconscious reactions.

A while ago, I created an infographic to help explain what safety might mean for us as individuals (see below). It would be easy to conclude that we feel 'safe' when there is an absence of threat – that makes logical sense – but in actual fact, that's only a small part of the story.

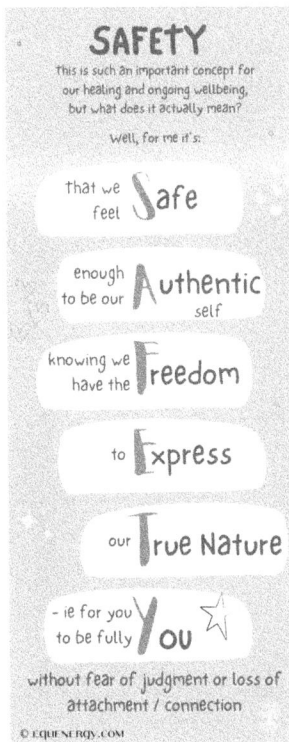

SAFETY

This is such an important concept for our healing and ongoing wellbeing, but what does it actually mean?

Well, for me it's:

that we feel **S**afe

enough to be our **A**uthentic self

knowing we have the **F**reedom

to **E**xpress

our **T**rue Nature

– ie for you to be fully **Y**ou

without fear of judgment or loss of attachment / connection

© EQUINERGY.COM

Consider this: you could be alone, or around people who present no threat or any intention of harm, and yet you might still be feeling on edge, anxious, or even fearful. In this scenario, the above summation of 'safe' being the absence of threat, doesn't work.

But why is this? Why do we have feelings of fear if there is no obvious threat?

The answer lies in our subconscious. Our subconscious doesn't necessarily care if the threat is real or not, it will happily pick up on something it perceives as a threat or if we are already in a state of hypervigilance, it might identify everything as a potential threat. And, when this happens (regardless of cause), our body goes straight into a (major) stress state where we will default into one of the 7 'F's: '**F**ight, **F**lee, **F**reeze, **F**awn, **F**ix, **F**lop or **F**idget'.

To help illustrate these 7 'F's', I've used animals (see image on next page) and included examples of how these behaviours could present:

- Fight – becoming defensive and starting an argument with someone.
- Flee – feeling the need to run away and hide from a situation.
- Freeze – that moment when you literally stop, unable to speak or to act.
- Fawn – stepping into the role of people pleaser.
- Fix – trying to sort out everyone's problems for them.
- Flop – just wanting to crawl back under the bedclothes because you don't have the energy to deal with the situation.
- Fidget – clicking a pen or jiggling a foot.

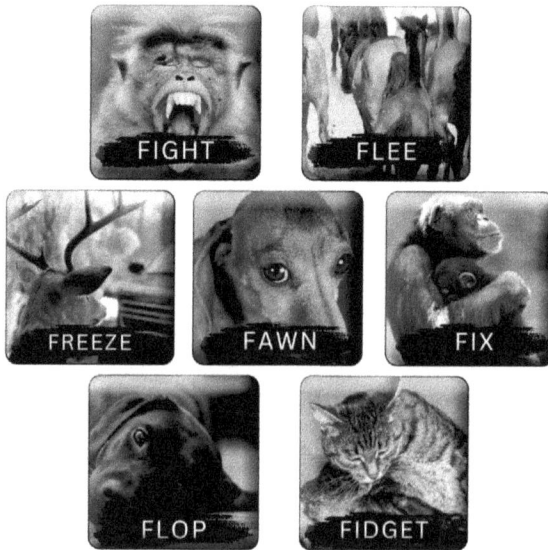

These are just some of the unconscious survival strategies we employ daily. What is important to realise is that we don't choose these survival strategies; they are automatic behaviours which become conditioned and habitual over time *until* we consciously decide to change them.

When we are in a place or feeling of 'safety,' we will experience the opposite of the 7 Fs. Our bodies will not go into a stress state, and we will find ourselves free from anxieties and fear, which is where we all want to be, right?

But – and this is key – we have to establish a sense of safety in order to move forward; it doesn't just 'happen' (the following pages will guide you on how to do this). If we don't establish this safety, then we could find our fearful and unhelpful behaviours/reactions increasing. And it can be challenging to achieve this sense of safety. We may still find ourselves reacting even when we've taken the time to create a safe space, which is because, when we explore things we've pushed down for so long, it can feel threatening. And don't forget, we pushed them down for a reason. They felt big, painful, scary and/or overwhelming, and we didn't know how to deal with them or cope with them, so we avoided them. (If you find this happening for you, it's good to reach out and ask for support, to find someone who can hold that sense of safety for you until you are able to do so for yourself.)

As children and adolescents, we may not have had a coping strategy for our fear, and even though we're adults now, inside of us, if we look really closely, we might still find that frightened child who felt so alone and didn't know how to handle such big emotions. Our inner critic often tries to diminish childhood fears and worries by telling us things like, 'Other people had it so much worse than you', or 'That was so long ago, and you're a grown-up now', or 'You should be able to handle this at your age' – but that is irrelevant. If our inner child still needs to feel safe and we have yet to develop this skill, we will be unable to process these emotions adequately as adults.

You might want to assess where you are at in terms of 'safety', in which case, a good place to start is to consider the following questions:

Do you feel safe in your physical environment?
This could be your home, your workplace, or anywhere you spend your time.

Do you feel safe in your relationships?
This could include your family, partner, work colleagues, or friends.

Do you feel safe with other people in general?
This could be either 1:1, in small groups, or in crowds.

Remember, this is about more than just physical safety, so if you've said 'Yes' to any of the categories above, don't forget to also answer these questions in terms of emotional and psychological safety.

If you answer 'No' to some or even all of the above, that is an indicator you need to create as much safety as you can for yourself. As a start, 'safety' might take the form of a place you can go to be completely comfortable and entirely yourself. Though a space is physical in its presence, spending time there can provide you with emotional and psychological safety too, by nature of its location perhaps, or the fact you don't have to pretend to be someone else when you are there. The place can be anywhere: a corner of your house, a greenhouse or shed, or maybe in your car or somewhere outdoors – it doesn't matter, as long as wherever you choose is somewhere you feel secure.

For me, there was a tree in a local park that I used to go to. It was growing at an angle, and I would lean against its trunk, feeling its strength, solidity and support behind my back and imagine its roots growing deep down into the ground. For a time, this tree was one of my favourite safe places.

Once you've found your place, think of what you can bring into it to enhance your feeling of safety. A nice warm blanket, a candle, a photo, some essential oils, or a plant, perhaps. Include all of your senses. Is there a piece of music which helps you to relax, for example? A perfume or a fragrant flower which brings back happy memories for you? Or is there a person, an animal or a place which helps you to feel safe? Perhaps you could put a photo of these in your safe place (if appropriate).

For the sense of touch, consider what textures help you feel comfortable, warm and relaxed. And taste/smell could be satisfied by a mug of your favourite tea, perhaps a relaxing herbal blend, or some water containing chopped fruit. As a personal example, the smell of baking bread and furniture polish always reminded me of happy times at my grandparents' house.

You can also create an 'anchor', which is basically associating how we want to feel with something tangible like a 'mudra' – a specific handshape – such as touching the tip of your index finger to the tip of your thumb on the same hand. You can also link (anchor) the associated feelings to a certain word, colour, scent, or piece of clothing. It could be your lucky belt, a pair of earrings, or a photo or image. If you have these, you can also include them on a vision board, which we will address in Chapter 5. If you have a strong imagination, you may be able to 'anchor' your feelings to a mental image.

◆ Exercise: Creating an 'Anchor'

Creating an anchor can be hugely beneficial and is easy to do if you follow these six simple steps:

1. Choose the feeling you want to anchor. In this instance, we are talking about safety.

2. Remember a time when you felt this way, i.e. a time when you felt totally safe.

> If you can't find a memory of a time when you felt safe, ask yourself: 'If I did experience that, though, how would it feel?' Do your best to imagine how it would feel for you.

3. Choose your anchor 'device'.

> For example, touching your thumb and forefinger together or stroking your upper arm with your hand

4. Remember what you saw, heard and felt in your memory of what it was like to be safe (or whatever feeling you are wishing to anchor).

5. Put numbers 3 and 4 together.

> Whilst employing your 'anchor' device, put yourself inside the memory as if reliving it here and now, in the present moment. Make it as real, bright and colourful an image as possible.

> You can also think of this as 're-membering' – returning this feeling of safety to part of the make-up of your being.

6. Practice.

> You may have to 'anchor' several times on different occasions before you can use the device on its own to achieve the desired feeling. But keep going. The more you practice, the more you are ingraining that feeling, and the easier your body will find it to respond in a positive way.

Repeating this exercise often throughout the day helps to strengthen the association between your chosen anchor and the feeling. Once it is ingrained, you can then bring the feeling to mind any time you want by using the anchor device.

Safety is also about whether or not we feel the deep sense of connection that we need in our lives. As human beings, we are social creatures, hard-wired to seek out connections of one form or another. These can be with other people, with animals, and with spaces, for example, your favourite park, the place where you grew up or where you currently live. I think of this connection as reflecting *our connection with ourselves* – our True Nature – a connection with our community, or 'our tribe' as it's often called, and a connection with the world around us. How we fit into the world and how we relate to the people we meet. If we fit in and are comfortable with how we relate to others, we will automatically have that connection and sense of safety.

Safety also requires compassion. As A H Almaas[2] says:

> *"It is only when compassion is present that people allow themselves to see the truth."*

When we feel this sense of safety, it begins to open us up to the Love that is Who We Really Are because there is no longer any fear around expressing our authentic Self—and we can own all aspects of our being. This part of us, our True Nature, always loves and supports us. When we begin to look at ourselves from this non-judgmental perspective, it allows us to experience deep self-compassion and connection. This, when it happens, is profoundly healing.

From this new perspective, this new space, if you like, we can see, appreciate, honour and witness our pain. I'm going to pause here for a moment to share an example simply because I know that some of these concepts can be difficult to understand and are easier to get your head around if you can apply them to a relatable example.

---

2   *Diamond Heart: Elements of the Real in Man - Page 85*

A colleague of mine recently asked me to meet with her. My mind immediately went to the worst-case scenario and started 'catastrophising', assuming that I was being summoned for a telling-off of some sort. It felt like being called to the headmaster's office, and I experienced a rising sense of panic and dread. But I recognised that this was all going on in my head and that the meeting might be nothing at all like the scenario I was imagining. So, I decided to get curious. I explored what I was feeling and where I'd felt this way before and realised I had slipped back into old fears of punishment, even when I hadn't done anything wrong. I saw myself as the child I had been, terrified of my dad's volatile moods.

Exploring my reaction in this way allowed me to feel deep compassion for my younger self, and (as an adult) I was able to appreciate the depth of her fear and realise I was still holding some of that in my body. This is what was being triggered again in the present, and now I understood, I could acknowledge the feeling (of fear at being called to a meeting) whilst also knowing that the fear was related to events from a long time ago and not to my current situation. I could then support myself to choose a different perspective, one which was open to a more productive outcome and that allowed me to approach the meeting with an open mind and a lighter heart.

As it turned out, my colleague just wanted to ask my opinion about something. Had I not gone through the process of unpicking my initial reaction, I would have wasted time and energy fretting and making myself miserable. Exploring our deep and uncomfortable emotions isn't easy, but the benefits are more than worth it.

There's a phrase which is often used in wellbeing circles, though I don't know who first said it:

'We need to feel it in order to heal it.'

Think about it. When we push our pain down, it doesn't go away. It's still there, active within us, slowly sapping our life force. However, if we are able to create a safe, compassionate, connected space, then it becomes possible to face the things that have felt Big, Complex, Painful and Scary and allow them to breathe. That way, we can converse with them and see them as teachers with something to share.

Simply sitting in our safe space gives us the opportunity to become still since there is no sense of threat, meaning we can relax. This allows us to recentre ourselves and our thoughts, which no longer need to be on the alert for danger. Spending time in stillness in our safe space can move us from a feeling of being scattered to a greater feeling of 'presence' in the moment. From here, it is easier to observe with greater objectivity and clarity.

When we've been in a state of hypervigilance, this stilling of our mind can feel alien at first, but with consistent practice, it gets easier, and eventually, we will be able to explore our situation with gentle curiosity and compassion. Also, when we feel safe and can connect with our inner stillness, it opens us up to hearing the 'nudgings' of our intuition. We may begin to see possibilities and opportunities where previously we saw only obstacles and hazards. We can also enter into a non-judgmental dialogue with ourselves to assess each option that presents itself, weighing up the advantages and disadvantages, considering the consequences and from this, drafting a plan of action. Remember to bear in mind that the aim is to keep a degree of flexibility to allow for unforeseen events. If we make sure to build in flexibility, we can benefit from a degree of resilience, which will enable us to bend with the unpredictable rather than for it to leave us feeling broken.

The more we practice this, the more we strengthen these neural pathways in our brain, and the more these feelings of safety, objectivity, clarity, curiosity, and compassion become our 'norm' or benchmark. We will more readily notice when we've moved away from this balance point, and we will have developed our knowledge of how to return to this state. Therefore, even though returning to our daily life, with its various challenges, might press our buttons and temporarily unbalance us, we will now have the tools to support ourselves back to a greater sense of agency and assurance. If we can get to this point where we are able to receive and accept this learning, that is where we find true and lasting healing.

Sometimes, this practice can be referred to as 'letting go', but I prefer Jack Kornfield's way of describing it – as 'letting be':

> "To let go does not mean to get rid of. To let go means to let be. When we let be with compassion, things come and go on their own."
> Jack Kornfield[3]

In order to create safety for yourself, you may feel the need to withdraw – temporarily, or in some cases permanently – from some of your previous relationships with people, places or activities, especially if they are triggering for you and make you feel threatened. Also, if these relationships are pushing you into those unconscious, conditioned behaviours we talked about at the beginning of the chapter (the 7 'F's), this may well be the validation you need to make that break.

This can be challenging and might be difficult for some of your family, friends, colleagues or acquaintances to accept – particularly if their relationship with you is one you are re-evaluating. They might try to convince you it's okay to stay as you were but remember there's a reason you started out on this journey. You're doing this for your wellbeing, which is the most important asset you have. Plus, you are worth it! No matter what anyone else might tell you, it's okay – and indeed proper – to put yourself first sometimes. Self-care is **not** selfish[4]. If we don't take good care of ourselves, we have nothing to give others. Our health, energy and goodwill will be eroded, leaving us feeling exhausted, frustrated, angry and probably ill. Engaging in (radical) self-care, and therefore role-modelling this to others, is one of the best gifts we can give ourselves and everyone else.

Trauma causes us to be disconnected; it triggers a chronic disruption of our connection (with the world and our Self). Healing, then, is a reversal of this disconnection, which is made possible through safety. When we feel safe, we can begin to come out of our shells, take off our armour, and return to our normal size. We can allow ourselves to be

---

3   *The Art Of Forgiveness, Loving Kindness And Peace, Jack Kornfield · 2010*
4   *To avoid this unfortunate association, self-care is therefore sometimes referred to as Inner Care. I mention this here in case you might find this a term you can more easily relate to.*

seen for who we are. Authenticity and vulnerability become possible because, with safety, we no longer feel judged or at risk of physical, verbal, emotional or psychological attack. This is why safety and how you recognise and achieve it is so important.

Think of it like a life jacket. In the water, we may be afraid, but with a life jacket, the fear is lessened or even removed. Safety (which we create or achieve) is the life jacket that supports our healing journey and ultimately enables us to be *Who We Really Are*.

In the previous chapter, I mentioned having 'someone in your corner' – either a trusted friend or a professional therapist/coach/mentor – which can be hugely beneficial. Remember, you don't have to do this alone; as I've said above, finding connection(s) is part of this journey. Having someone you can talk to and trust, who won't judge or even tell you what you 'should' do, can make all the difference. Someone who will hold space for you when you need it, reflect and mirror your experiences so that you can truly witness and acknowledge them and their impact on your life, and support you in finding the answers that are right for you will benefit you immensely.

There are many different practitioners and approaches out there, so feel free to take your time in finding one that's a good fit for you. If you're not sure where to start, then you might like to take a look at my blog: *7 Tips For Finding The Practitioner Who's Right For You ~ (https://www.equenergy.com/7-tips-for-finding-the-practitioner-whos-right-for-you/).*

As you start out on your W·I·L·D ® journey, I'd like you to check in with yourself - you could even do a sway test to help you (see page 142).

Ask:

- How safe do I feel right now – physically, emotionally, and psychologically?
- Can I give this a number out of 10 or a percentage?

Make a note of your answers because if they have shown that you don't feel safe in any one or a combination of the aspects listed above, or if you get a low number or percentage, then now is the time to address this, even before moving on to the following chapters. It's never too early - or too late - to put safety in place for ourselves or address areas of our lives where we don't feel safe. It's about laying a good foundation for what we want to build going forward.

In summary, safety is key.

You can find some free resources on my YouTube channel *(https://www.youtube.com/@W-I-L-D-TV)* in the Self-Care Exercises playlist.

(If you'd like to explore further how to create a sense of safety for yourself along with tools that you can use for support, you'll find several modules in my Create Your Own W·I·L·D® Wellbeing learning programme, which will assist you. The programme is available on my website (www.equenergy.com) under the 'Working with me' tab. There's a wide range of options, so you can pick and choose to tailor-make a programme that works for you and your budget.)

Chapter Summary

We:

- Looked at the essential concept of Safety and learned how this underpins any wellbeing or healing journey. Unless we can create a sense of safety for ourselves, we will not be able to release our fears, reach out for support, or process the traumas and hurts that are currently holding us in the repeating patterns that have contributed to our current situation.
- Explored ways to figure out how to feel safe and learned that it is an ongoing process which will continually evolve.
- Understood that self-care is not selfish. It is, in fact, one of the most generous things we can do for those around us as well as ourselves. If we prefer, we can use the alternative term inner care.

~ Four ~
The W·I·L·D® Way

Inside Chapter Four

Here, we will delve further into the concept of W·I·L·D®, giving us an appreciation of our bodies as the wonder-full, intelligent, bio-logical systems they are. We will gain a deeper understanding of how and why they respond to the stresses we experience in our lives and learn that contrary to what we might think, they are not going wrong, making a mistake or attacking us. Our bodies are simply making adaptations which, despite outward appearances, are not random. On some level, these adaptations or changes have a purpose and it's in uncovering these that we learn how to best support true and lasting healing.

~ ~ ~ ~ ~

Over the years, W•I•L•D® Wellbeing has grown and evolved organically, and along the way, I have adjusted – particularly in branding as I've become clearer in my focus. Part of this change has seen the creation of my W·I·L·D® acronym, which I went on to register as a trademark in early 2023. It has felt like quite a long gestation and birthing process to get to this point however with the solidifying of W·I·L·D®, my work feels more deeply rooted than ever, which is partly what has led me to write this book now.

Nature – as I have mentioned before - has been such a huge force and presence in my healing adventure. She has taught me so much and been my constant guide, confidant and cheerleader along the way, so it was only natural for the W·I·L·D® acronym to reflect this. Life can get messy – as can Nature – and W·I·L·D® both reflects and celebrates this.

So often, as humans, we want things to be neat and tidy, to fall within prescribed boundaries and follow the rules, but Nature follows her own rules! She colours outside of the lines. She shakes things up. Her winds roar; her sun shines with fierce heat; her tides crash with enough power to split rock. And yet she can be as gentle as a soft breeze or a tender rain. She can be vast, like space, or tiny, like a single-celled organism. She comes in all kinds of shapes, sizes and colours, with infinite variety. She's full of beautiful patterns and repetition, and yet each individual is unique. She ebbs and flows with seasons, tides, days and nights. She provides us with food to eat, water to drink, and shelter to keep us safe and warm. She is our nurturing Mother and the teacher who knows the most effective way to challenge and bring out the best in us.

Humans often think we can do better than Nature and that we aren't governed by her laws, but when we disconnect from the laws of Mother Nature and stray too far into our brain-dominated ways, it tends to lead to problems. This is because when we allow our brains to dominate, we lose the balancing influences of our heart and gut. Nature is a bio-logical[1], intelligent system – just like our bodies - which is designed to function interdependently. It seeks to be in balance – or, as I tend to think of it, balance-ing (as a verb rather than a noun); a dynamic, changing, responsive action rather than a 'once and done' static deed. And just as our bodies can experience dis-ease, so too can Nature.

We don't have to look too far to find examples of this, such as the volume of plastic[2] and microplastics[3] in the oceans and the impact of glyphosate weed killers on our bee populations. But Nature, too, can heal, and I would definitely recommend following the link to this video.

---

1   *This is another word which I split to highlight the way in which I use it. There is a logical reason and purpose to the way things work in Nature. We might think that processes are random, whereas, in fact, they follow clear natural laws and systems.*
2   *For example, turtles find it difficult to differentiate between plastic bags and jellyfish and autopsies on marine animals who have been found dead or emaciated have revealed that their stomachs have been full of plastic.*
3   *As plastics degrade and become microplastics, their chemical components can leach into their surroundings, including living tissue. A large number of these chemicals (2,400 of them) have been classified as substances of potential concern, meeting the European Union's criteria for persistence, bioaccumulation, or toxicity. For example, many of them act as endocrine-disrupting compounds, or toxicants that imitate hormones when they enter the body. Hormones are active at very low concentrations in the bloodstream and as some chemical additives in plastic resemble hormones, the body responds. They might also cause other problems such as inflammatory responses. (https:// www.webmd.com/a-to-z-guides/news/20221028/microplastics-health-risks-what-do-we-really-know)*

(If you're reading the print book or are not using a multi-media device, then you'll need to make a note of the address for later).

It is a beautiful illustration of how Nature can be restored; in this particular situation, it is the result of reintroducing wolves which changed the course of rivers in Yellowstone National Park in America *(https://www.youtube.com/watch?v=ysa5OBhXz-Q&t=69s)*.

We sometimes forget that humans are animals, too, and that we have mammalian instincts and responses. Society may try to tell us otherwise and condition us into believing that we've left those parts of ourselves behind in our cave-dwelling past, but in fact, they're still very active and play a large part in our wellbeing—but only when we provide them with the resources and freedom they need to do so.

W·I·L·D®, then, is an acknowledgement that, just like our domesticated cats and dogs, there remains a 'wild-ness' within us, that deep connection with Nature. We still respond to the rhythms of day and night (circadian rhythm), the cycles of the moon and of the seasons. Our bodies experience cravings for certain foods because they know what they need at that time, and we are still captives of automatic responses such as fight, flight, freeze and flop. These are part of our inbuilt animal survival mechanisms, and although we might not have to fight predators on a regular basis anymore, these strategies are present and active within us. Ignoring them doesn't mean that they go away; in fact, if we choose not to acknowledge them, not to find expression for them, they will remain held within our bodies. The choice to ignore them may be an active decision, or it might be arrived at through our conditioning, but if we don't allow them space, they can and will lead to dis-ease.

Giving ourselves permission to reconnect with our wildness and to find appropriate ways of expressing the emotions and responses that it brings up supports our wellbeing. Through express-ion, we can 'get it all out' so that the emotions are no longer held inside of us, festering away and potentially making us sick. As best-selling author Bessel van der Kolk explains in his book, '*The Body Keeps the Score*', our 'body does not forget'. What he means by this is that our bodies retain everything in order that we can continue to learn and grow; however, if we don't allow the resulting emotions out, that's when we internalise, and that can be hugely damaging.

There's a great quote from the writer and spiritual teacher A H Almaas:

"Your conflicts, all the difficult things, the problematic situations in your life are not chance or haphazard; they're actually yours. They're specifically yours, designed specifically for you, by the part of you that loves you more than anything else. The part of you that loves you more than anything else has created roadblocks to lead you to yourself. You're not going to go in the right direction unless there's something pricking you in the side telling you, look here, this way. That part of you loves you so much that it won't let you lose the chance. It will go to extreme measures to wake you up. It will make you suffer greatly if you don't listen. What else can it do? That's its purpose."

Nature is always seeking our survival. Even more than this, she wants us to thrive because when we're thriving, we're growing and learning, we're nurturing offspring, and we're passing what we've learnt onto them so that the process continues.

Take the example of a plant. If it's sickly, it won't flower and bear fruit. It needs to have the right conditions in order to be healthy and create future generations (fruit) - we are the same. We need the right conditions in order to thrive and grow. We need an optimum environment and the exact amount of light, food and water – both literally and metaphorically. We gain these conditions from what we ingest, i.e. the food we eat, what we read, watch and listen to, the people we spend time with and the conversations we engage in. Our environment is also affected by how we choose to perceive the world in which we live, which brings us back to the **thought-belief cycle** we discussed earlier. (See page 67 to refresh your memory).

You might find it strange when I say how we 'choose' to perceive the world, particularly as this isn't something we (usually) consciously choose. Generally, we believe that our perception of the world is based on what we have seen and how things are, but from what I've shared thus far and what you will learn as we go through the stages of W·I·L·D® you will start to understand that in actual fact, it's not that simple.

This quote sums it up perfectly (source unknown):

*"We don't see things as **they** are; we see them as **we** are."*

We all see the world differently, and how we see it and perceive our place in it can have a direct impact on our wellbeing. If we start to experience symptoms of dis-ease, then it's helpful to tune in to our body and 'ask' what wisdom it's seeking to share with us. It could well be that our interpretation of the situation - as opposed to its reality - is contributing to our dis-ease. To check this, you can ask yourself questions such as:

- What emotions/responses am I holding that I haven't felt able to express?
- What beliefs come from this, or what beliefs are causing my reaction?
- What are the underlying, currently unmet needs, and how might I meet these in appropriate and supportive ways?

I believe that symptoms, in fact, every feeling that we experience, are just communication. Our body simply wants to tell us something, and, as it has no voice, it shows us by how we feel. It's a kind of body 'vocabulary' that we can tune into and learn to build up a dialogue and an understanding.

One effective way to tune into our bodies is to use a Body Scan. My YouTube channel has an example of this at *https://equenergy.com/BodyScan/.*

Once you've completed a body scan (or similar), you should have an increased awareness of the sensations within your body. It is helpful to repeat this exercise regularly as it takes practice to tune in and listen, so the more frequently you undertake such an exercise, the easier it will become to find and identify these sensations. Once you have identified them, you can now view them in a different way. Hopefully, you will learn to appreciate they are not something to be afraid of; in fact, they are to be welcomed because they will help us to learn more about ourselves and how best to support our wellbeing.

Seeing dis-ease as a valuable teacher might sound like an odd way of looking at things, and years ago, I'd have thought it was completely bizarre, too, simply because it didn't fit with what I'd learnt up until that point. I believed the truth to be what I'd been taught in school, and anything that I read and absorbed was 'right'. To be honest, I never really questioned anything until I began my journey of healing, but now my perspective has changed dramatically. Through learning and going deeper into my own various ills, I'm much more likely to explore rather than take things as read and to 'test out' theories and ask questions.

At first, this new perspective on dis-ease felt very odd, even uncomfortable. It meant I had to leave behind my 'certainties' and step out into the unknown. Brené Brown calls this going out into the 'wilderness', and it should not be underestimated how deeply challenging this can be. As humans, we have the desire to connect and to 'belong', which we've come to see as 'fitting in', but Brené Brown, in exploring Maya Angelou's quote,

> *"You only are free when you realise you belong no place — you belong every place — no place at all,"*

says that if 'fitting in' means suppressing our True Nature in order to 'conform', then this is the opposite of belonging[4]. Brené Brown goes on to comment that this will leave us feeling even more disconnected than before because by 'fitting in' (with the majority), we will have disconnected from our true Self – and this is the cause of the deepest of all wounds.

---

4 *Braving the Wilderness, Brené Brown*

W·I·L·D® looks at how we can address this, how we can get curious about what we're feeling and respond to the communications from our body. It's about how we can balance our need to feel that deep connection with Self whilst at the same time creating a sense of safety and belonging – to ourselves and to Nature – so that we can start to feel comfortable in our own skin. Then we can truly in-joy (that is, 'bring joy into') this experience of Life whilst also sharing the very best of ourselves with the world.

Over the next four chapters, I will take you through each letter of the acronym in turn so that you can begin your very own W·I·L·D® journey.

Good luck and enjoy!

Chapter Summary

- We acknowledged our bodies as the bio-logical systems they are and began to understand how they work for us (not against us) and seek to support our survival.

- I shared a Body Scan practice and some Self-Care Exercises for you to explore and add to your wellbeing toolkit. Remember to revisit these from time to time, as you might find that different things work for you at different times and in different situations as your needs change and evolve.

~ Five ~

W·I·L·D®
W is for Wonder

Inside Chapter Five

In this chapter, we'll be exploring the 'W' of W·I·L·D®, which stands for Wonder. Wonder encompasses how we look at the world around us and how this, in turn, impacts our sense of Self and wellbeing. We will consider how you are currently viewing yourself and your situation, whether it is serving you, and decide how you would like your life to feel and whether your current perspective is in line with this. And if not, how might you make a shift?

~ ~ ~ ~ ~

As I began to appreciate more fully the truth of that quote: *"We don't see things as they are; we see them as WE are,"* I started to explore my own thoughts, beliefs and perceptions and examine how these might have been colouring my experiences. You can liken this process to cleaning your glasses. When you realise they are dirty, you'll know that they have been making your world appear darker and grimier than it really is. When you clean them, the world changes for the better; indeed, it becomes full of Wonder, which is what I discovered as I started to explore my thoughts, beliefs and perceptions. Turns out my 'glasses' really did need a good clean!

As you might have noticed, I love quotes. I find they often encapsulate things beautifully and succinctly, so I'd like to share another couple here which have had a huge impact:

*"When you change the way you look at things,
the things you look at change."*
Wayne Dyer

and

*"The moment you change your perception, is the
moment you rewrite the chemistry of your body."*
Bruce Lipton

Both of these are short and, at first glance, appear deceptively simple, but sit for a moment with each of them in turn and think about what they would actually mean for your life.

I came across Wayne Dyer's words first. At the time I would fret when people didn't quickly reply to my texts or emails. I would automatically assume that I had upset them in some way or that they had decided they no longer wished to connect with me. My old fears of abandonment and rejection would resurface, leaving me feeling hurt, upset and isolated. When I found Wayne Dyer's words, though, I took a moment to think about them and suddenly, things made much more sense. I finally understood that my perception was determining how the world appeared to me – and that because it was mine, it was within my control. I could change it. I could choose how to look at things. I realised that I could choose to continue seeing my world negatively, feeling that everything was against me and that my life was miserable and deeply unfair… or I could find another way that felt better.

I applied this new thought process to the example above, where I worried if people didn't reply to my texts or emails and, when I did, I realised it was nothing to do with me at all. The reality was that those I was texting and emailing were simply busy and caught up in their own lives and their lack of prompt response was in no way a reflection on me. In fact, I took it a stage further. I opened my thinking and allowed myself to really dig into this being my issue as opposed to the person I was contacting.

And that was when it dawned on me. **I wasn't that important**.

That's not a negative comment—far from it. It simply means I believed myself to be so important in their lives that if they didn't respond as I thought they should, it meant they no longer wished to be associated with me. Yet, in actuality, we are never that important to anyone other than ourselves. Initially, this might sound harsh, but in fact, it is liberating.

To further illustrate this point, whenever I would receive a message from someone asking to meet with me, I would automatically assume that they were angry with me and that I was about to be punished, but again, this was my perception rather than the truth, and once I understood that I began to find dealing with these scenarios a lot easier.

Sadly, it can be common for people to go straight to these 'worst case scenarios' without even considering the many other possibilities that are more likely to be true. When I later read Dr Lipton's words (*"The moment you change your perception, is the moment you rewrite the chemistry of your body"*), it was like the final missing puzzle piece. His use of the word 'chemistry' immediately made me realise how my perception(s) affected my body and, thus, my wellbeing. Putting these two quotes together, I could see that by changing my perception, I could change my body and ultimately create a healthier inner environment.

Dr Lipton[1] teaches that it's not the genes we're born with which determine our state of health, but how those genes express themselves (i.e. how they switch on and off), and we can influence this by the choices we make: our thoughts, beliefs, and the environment that we create for ourselves (what we eat, how we move, what we listen to, the people we spend time with, etc.). I've mentioned that once I understood 'things were within my control,' it was a profound and life-changing moment. It might sound obvious, but for me, this was huge.

Up until that point, I hadn't realised that I had this power, this choice.

---

1   *The Biology of Belief, Bruce Lipton Ph.D*

On the surface, yes, I had as many options as the next person, but did I feel able to choose?

Not so much.

But the question here is, why not?

The answer was blindingly simple. Because I had become a people pleaser. I was afraid to rock the boat. I wanted to fit in (that human need), so I went along with other people's decisions. I let people at work walk all over me. I suppressed my feelings, gritted my teeth, put my head down and got on with it. But these actions were making me sick (though I had no idea). These were behaviours I'd learnt in childhood as a survival strategy in the face of my dad's volatile temper. When I later encountered a boss who reminded me of my father, it brought out that inner frightened child, and I slipped right back into those old behaviours again. People pleasing. Agreeing to go along with the crowd.

When I finally handed in my notice and left that job (even though I still worked there on a freelance basis), it gave me sufficient space to see what had been happening, and that's when I was able to take back some of my power to choose.

As I said back in Chapter 2, I'd become fascinated by energy early on in my journey, and by now, I had discovered that different emotions have different 'vibrations'. (See the diagram opposite.) In addition, I discovered Abraham-Hicks' teachings, such as the book 'The Law of Attraction – The Basics of the Teachings of Abraham', as well as 'The Secret' by Rhonda Byrne, where she shares her teachings on the art of manifestation. I came to understand that joy/gratitude is one of the highest vibrations we can experience and that higher vibrations are incredibly healing – not only to ourselves internally but also to the outside world. Energy is 'contagious' and, therefore, readily shared with those around us.

Until I started to really understand energy and its impact, I had been experiencing little to no joy in my life, and I certainly wasn't feeling

THE EMOTION SCALE

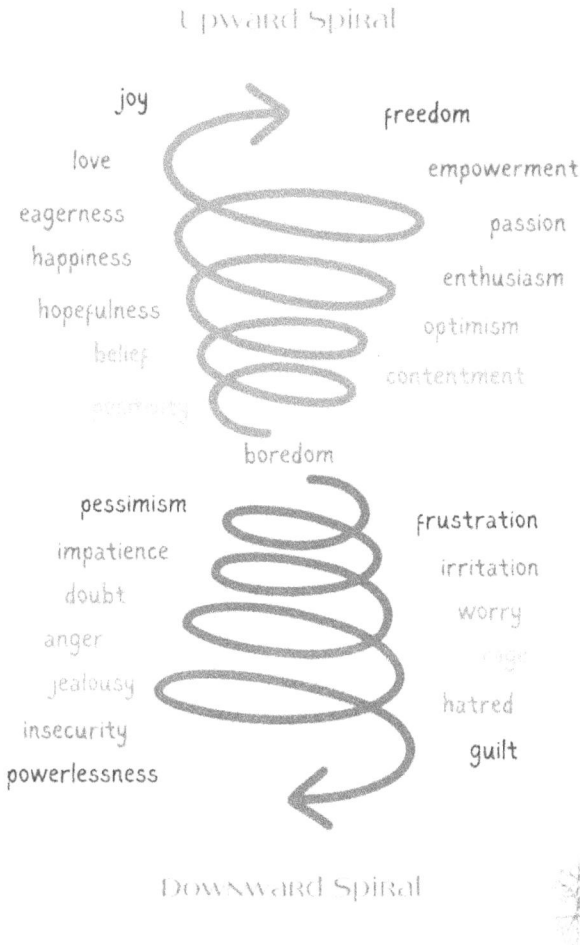

Upward Spiral

joy

freedom

love

empowerment

eagerness

passion

happiness

enthusiasm

hopefulness

optimism

belief

contentment

boredom

pessimism

frustration

impatience

irritation

doubt

worry

anger

jealousy

hatred

insecurity

guilt

powerlessness

Downward Spiral

very grateful. In hindsight, it was no wonder that my health had been deteriorating - but then, how could I possibly feel joyful or grateful when my life seemed so miserable? This is where I was stuck. You may well have experienced something similar or may even be stuck there right now. It's all well and good saying that changing our energy positively will impact us positively, but if we feel there is nothing to be happy about, how on earth would we achieve this?

It was at this point I remembered Wayne Dyer's words:

"The moment you change the way you look at things, the things you look at change."

And I began to Wonder (the 'W' in W·I·L·D ®), could this really be true? Could it be that simple? Could my life change for the better simply because I altered my perspective?

I was incredibly sceptical. Changing my perspective would mean changing the beliefs I'd held for years, and whether or not I tried to make that change started to feel like a way to test my determination to heal. If I were truly committed to healing, then I would make the change, but if I wasn't …

I was also stuck in the loop of believing that my long-held belief system provided me with the safety I needed to continue in life, so the question became: was I committed enough to give up the beliefs and biases that I was convinced had held me safe thus far? Committed enough to accept I'd been (potentially) getting it wrong all these years? Committed enough to open myself up to feeling foolish?

There was no question. Yes. Absolutely.

I had reached the point where what I had to lose was less than what I could potentially gain. It was a no-brainer.

But I had no idea how to start, so I began asking myself some questions (which can be a great place for you to start as well).

I asked:

- Where had I developed these perceptions? In particular, why did I believe that my life was so rotten and unfair, and were these perceptions actually correct?
- What might life look like if I changed this perspective, and how could I get myself to that new viewpoint?

One thing I was certain of was that I wouldn't be able to 'fake' this. I had to go all in and truly believe that I could instigate such changes. If I didn't, I knew that I'd see right through my efforts and lose any sense of trust in myself, so this had to be real.

In my reading, I'd also come across another concept:

"Everyone is doing the best they can with the resources they have available to them in that moment."[2]

Yet I wasn't sure I believed this for myself. Was I really doing the best I could with the resources I had available?

My inner critic jumped straight in and told me that I wasn't. It tried to convince me I could be mean and horrible sometimes, which surely wasn't me at my best. Though that voice was tough to ignore, I had come to learn its narrative wasn't always faithful and that it often repeated the words of others, which I had taken in and accepted as 'truth'—but what if they weren't true? How mind-blowing would that be?

Our inner critic uses these words as its own means of keeping us 'safe'. **And this is a key point**. Our critic genuinely believes that these words, which have led to our 'faulty' beliefs, have kept us alive thus far and so reminds us of them at every opportunity. The reality is that this is simply not true.

Remember, our inner critic recycles messages it has heard from others, which are based on their belief systems, not ours. Where the messages cause us discomfort, this is evidence that they are not true for us.

Challenging my inner critic was far from easy, so don't worry if you struggle with this at first. But what I realised was that the more I questioned that voice, the more I was able to reassure it that its beliefs were faulty and misplaced. Once I began to really understand this, the (re)educating of my inner voice became my first focus.

I began to challenge this voice by telling it that everything was okay and I'd 'got this'.

---

2 For example, in Brené Brown's book, *Braving The Wilderness*

(Some people give their inner voices a name or identity at this stage. It can be easier to converse with when it has its own separate identity.)

The next logical step was to take a good, hard look at my old thought patterns and consider suspending them. Note that I've used the word 'suspended' here. Rather than telling these thoughts that they were 'wrong' or 'bad', I simply wanted to explore an alternative to see if it might feel better. In this way, I felt that any change would be less likely to feel threatening or overwhelming.

The first thought pattern/belief system I suspended was the one of judgement of others. Previously, I had based this on my personal thought-belief system, but instead, I chose to accept they were 'simply doing the best they could [from their perspective] with the tools available to them at the time'. In other words, I started to give everyone the 'benefit of the doubt' until I had reason not to.

It seemed a small adjustment, and I was unsure what difference it would make, but I knew I had to start with something achievable, and that felt like a good place to begin. To my surprise, it made much more of a difference than I ever imagined. Not only did it enable me to become more compassionate towards others, but it also took the pressure off me to be 'perfect'. I gave myself the same 'pass' I gave others, which led to me becoming much more relaxed.

> **TIP:** I recommend trying this yourself. When you are looking at the world, at others and viewing them/it in a negative light, try reminding yourself that we are all just doing the best we can, and keep telling yourself that to reinforce it. See what a change it can make for you.

Several times along this journey, I've discovered that seemingly small and simple changes can have a huge impact, which has led me to conclude that we view our problems as Big, Complex, Painful and Scary, so we assume that the answers must also be Big, Complex, Painful and Scary. Yet, **spoiler alert**, this isn't the case most of the time – if ever. The answers can often be found in simple solutions that we may initially dismiss as being too small and/or too simple. In fact,

I would go further and say that in my experience, keeping it small, simple and straightforward (KISSS) is the key. Looking at my journey in small, achievable steps has made it feel much more manageable and, therefore, easier to keep moving forward with.

The reason for KISSS is sound: When we keep it simple, we don't feel as if we've 'bitten off more than we can chew', and thus, the situation/issue no longer feels so overwhelming.

Note: If you're someone who experienced childhood trauma, then overwhelm can easily rear its ugly head. Remembering KISSS can make this process feel much less threatening meaning it is less likely to reactivate the fear that our body carries from that early trauma.

I started putting these new perceptions into practice, remembering to find things to be grateful for and – as Brené Brown calls it in her book *Braving the Wilderness* - being 'generous' in my 'interpretation of other people's motivations' and doing my 'best to see them in a positive light'.

This felt significantly different to how I was looking at things previously.

If we refer again to the **thought-belief cycle** (reshared on the next page), this can be a helpful illustrator. Imagine, for a moment, that you are going to insert 'low vibration' thoughts into this cycle (for clarification of low and high vibration thoughts, see the illustration below the cycle).

Inserting a low-vibration thought will lead to beliefs with a negative bias, which will give our perspective a more pessimistic slant. The filters we then use come from a place of challenge and uncertainty, and therefore, the meaning we attribute to how we are feeling and the experiences we have will also be primarily negatively focused.

Now, change that initial low-vibration thought to a high-vibration one.

See the difference?

THE THOUGHT-BELIEF CYCLE

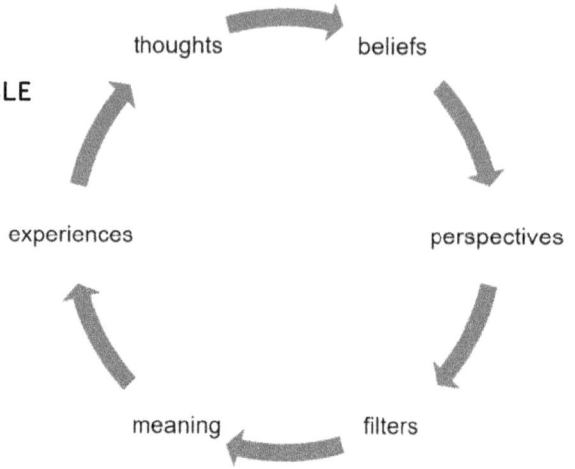

thoughts → beliefs → perspectives → filters → meaning → experiences → thoughts

THE EMOTION SCALE

Upward Spiral

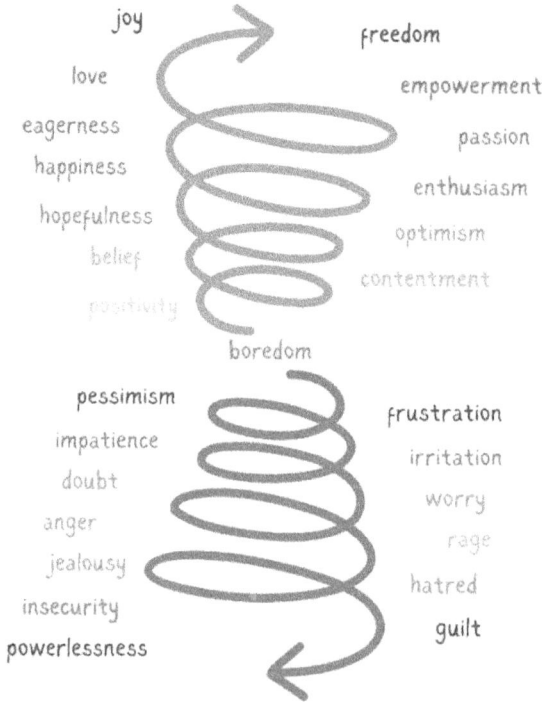

joy
freedom
love
empowerment
eagerness
passion
happiness
enthusiasm
hopefulness
optimism
belief
contentment
positivity

boredom

pessimism
frustration
impatience
irritation
doubt
worry
anger
rage
jealousy
hatred
insecurity
guilt
powerlessness

Downward Spiral

As I continued to become more generous with myself and others, slowly, my world gained colour and light. It was as if I'd wiped my metaphorical 'glasses' and was seeing things with clarity for the first time in years. It felt liberating! I even had moments of laughter, which had long been missing from my life. It was wonder-full!

I took that feeling of Wonder and ran with it because, by definition, Wonder is to be curious and ask questions, but the premise of Wonder is also to experience joy. Both definitions fit exactly how I was feeling and what I was discovering, which is how Wonder came to be the first letter of W·I·L·D®.

Wonder is very experiential. You may have heard it said that we have a 'head brain', a 'heart brain', and a 'gut brain', which are 'interconnected and interdependent' and designed to 'work together in balance and harmony'. In our Newtonian[3], mechanistic society, however, we have sought to divide these and have given much more weight and respect to the head brain, often leaving the heart and gut brains as an afterthought.

If you think about our education system here in the UK, it is a great example of what I mean. Our system focuses heavily on 'left-brained' learning and qualifications (highly structured facts and figures) as opposed to more 'right-brained' pursuits (creative, colourful and artistic). Whilst there are undoubtedly some exceptions to this rule, and people are (in many circles) actively trying to redress this imbalance, left-brained thinking is still the predominant bias in our educational system and by extension, our society.

From my learnings, I have come to believe that for us to experience true and lasting healing, we will all benefit from becoming more balanced by aligning our left and right-side brains more closely. How, though, can we do this when some of us are born to be naturally methodical, highly organised, and intelligent, whilst others are more creative and have a greater ability to think outside the box and explore different ideas?

---

3   *That is, relating to or arising from the work of Sir Isaac Newton, basing beliefs on the principles of classical physics.*

In my workshop *In-Joy Your Life – the W·I·L·D® Way*, I share some exercises to help build your 'body vocabulary', that is, understanding how our body communicates with us through our physical and emotional sensations so that we can begin to establish a dialogue. Our bodies are constantly sending us messages, starting with a quiet whisper, but if we aren't listening or we're not able to hear or understand these messages, it will begin to 'shout' because it has no other option. 'Shouting' will manifest in pain and dis-ease, anxiety and stress, for example, and is our body's way of telling us that we need to pay attention and address the issues (it is highlighting) so that we can begin to heal. Our body has a blueprint of how it should look when functioning at its optimum and has all the processes it needs to get back to this, providing we give it the right environment and adequate resources. When we learn how to listen and respond, our body feels heard, and it can turn down its volume once again.

The first step here is to *learn* how to tune in and listen to our body, and to achieve this we need to get to know our body. Think of it like a new relationship where you are spending time getting to know the other person. Discover and understand what your body likes and dislikes, what its preferences are and what makes it tick. It will 'speak' to you in the form of physical sensations, posture and emotions, and these are what we must listen to.

I believe it's important to learn how our body shows us it is unhappy/stressed and, equally, how we know that it's contented/relaxed. This can be a very individual thing. There will be areas of overlap from person to person, but we also have our own unique list of what feels 'good' for us versus what feels 'off'. To support people in taking this first step, I usually suggest trying the Body Scan exercise that I mentioned in the previous chapter. It is a really useful resource and can help you to dig deep into the language of your body. (You can find this at *https://equenergy.com/BodyScan.*)

Repeating this exercise from time to time throughout your day/week will increase your understanding of your body and the sensations and emotions it shares with you. You can then start to observe which of these relate to stress and which feel supportive and uplifting.

◆ Exercise: How does it feel to be in 'Stress' vs in 'Flow'?

I invite you to pause your reading at this point and try the following:

- Take a piece of paper and draw a line down the middle from top to bottom, dividing the page into two halves.
- On one side, write the title 'stressed' – or whatever term feels appropriate for you. On the other side write something like 'ease' or 'flow' – whatever word best represents those supportive, uplifting feelings for you.
- Now, make a list under each heading of the emotions and physical sensations that belong in that category for you. *(You might like to refer to the Emotion Wheel in Appendix 6 for ideas on feelings to include in your lists.)* This is the start of your body's personal vocabulary and can help you gain greater clarity around what you're feeling and what it means for you.

   Some common examples are:
   ~ when stressed, we might feel anxious, insecure and/or worthless.
   ~ when at ease, we could feel relaxed, happy and/or hopeful

- Then, once you have these lists, try to use this 'vocabulary' regularly, whether that be via journaling or simply taking a moment to listen to your body and note how you are feeling. The more you use these words/emotions and attribute them to your body, the easier it will become to spot patterns in your responses and observe which feelings come up and when. You can then see if certain emotions appear at the same trigger points, i.e. related to specific people or situations, places or times.

This exercise is a great way to recognise areas of challenge and where you could benefit from some extra support or self-care. It can also assist you in identifying the types of things you can do to help yourself feel better.

Once you've got the hang of it, you can narrow down your exploration to find things specific to emotions on the higher end of the vibrational spectrum, for example. This includes emotions like joy, gratitude and wonder, which for me, I experience by:

◊   watching a sunset
◊   looking at the moon, the stars or the ocean
◊   contemplating an ancient tree
◊   examining the intricacies of a leaf
◊   or, as I discovered when I moved here, staring in awe at the beauty of the underside of a dung beetle!

You'll notice, perhaps unsurprisingly, that my examples come from Nature. Yours might be very different, and that's okay. In fact, it's wonder-full! My husband (as an engineer) gets enthralled by the beauty of engineering, so he experiences joy, gratitude, and wonder when looking at the design of a bridge or a beautifully machined tool or engine component. Try to take some time to discover your own list of experiences, places or people that generate those higher vibrating emotions in you. You will then be able to go straight to these activities/places/people, etc... when you need to move your emotions up the vibrational spectrum.

One thing to bear in mind is that our emotional triggers change over time, so it can be good to review yours and this exercise regularly. If you find one of your 'higher vibrational' activities is not currently feeling supportive, this can be a good indicator that it's time to refresh your practice and begin exploring some other options.

When it comes to a sense of Wonder, I personally feel this relates to the spiritual aspect of our being - not necessarily related to religion, but I believe we all have a part of our being that longs for the spiritual in some shape or form. Spiritual can be difficult to define, so I was delighted to come across this quote some time ago:

"A spiritual practice is anything that makes you feel
more beautiful inside you."
(Sri Avinash Do)

I think this is true. If you take time to consider what makes you feel more beautiful inside, arguably, you will be discovering a spiritual aspect of your being.

I've also heard spirituality described as a 'connection', which I interpret as a connection to our True Nature, to those around us, and/or to something bigger than ourselves. A force, if you like, that joins us all together – a kind of Life Force Energy – which is actually where the term Reiki comes from (Rei-Life force, Ki-energy).

In modern society, we can so often be in our own 'headspace' trying to analyse, rationalise and make sense of the world - effectively attempting to fit ourselves neatly into boxes, compartments or pigeonholes. But, like Nature, Life doesn't always remain within the lines. It can appear messy and 'untamed' – you could say it is W·I·L·D®.

Robert Bly sums it up:

> *"To be wild is not to be crazy or psychotic.*
> *True wildness is a love of Nature,*
> *a delight in silence,*
> *a voice free to say spontaneous things,*
> *and an exuberant curiosity in the face of the unknown."*

These few lines so aptly encapsulate Joy and Wonder. A true 'joie de vivre' – Joy of Life – where we're not simply 'existing' or 'surviving' but truly revelling in Life, engaging with it, putting in and taking out as much as possible. 'In-joy-ing' (bringing joy into) every experience and extracting as much learning and pleasure as possible.

I learnt during my research, our hearts produce more electromagnetic activity than our brains – which, if you think of all the neurons that are constantly firing in our brains, is pretty impressive. In addition, I also discovered that our gut sends more messages to our brains than our brains send down to our guts, so why do we often think that our 'head brain' is more important than the feedback we get from our body? If you break this simple fact down, our guts are definitely calling the shots.

Take a moment to re-read that paragraph and really consider this. We always emphasise (and believe and buy into) the messages our brain sends, the thought and logic messages, yet physiologically, our gut sends way more messages to our brain than the other way around. If you then add in another physiological fact, that our hearts are producing more electromagnetic energy than our brains, suddenly you can start to see the sense in listening more to our hearts and guts than to our 'head brain'.

◆ Exercise: Listening to the Wisdom of your Heart and Gut

Really allow yourself to observe and feel the communication between your gut and your brain and then between your heart and your brain. Ask yourself what messages your gut is sending to your brain. What messages is your heart sending to your brain?

These messages might be physical symptoms or emotions rather than thoughts and sensations, and that's great. It doesn't matter what form the messages take. The key is simply to notice them and write them down because your brain is being sent these messages for a reason.

As you progress through this book, I recommend you take time often to pause, reflect, and notice. Decide what part of your body is speaking to you and listen to what it is saying. Again, note this down. You may feel uncertainty, discomfort, or disagreement, but don't stop listening, no matter how challenging. All of these feelings hold some kind of wisdom.

Wonder then, if taken alongside our inner feelings and sense of spirit, will bring us back into connection with our body, our heart and our gut - those three wonderful communicators and teachers. So now it's time to put this into practice.

◆ Exercise: Somatic Journaling

I invite you to take a few moments here to pause and engage in a short exercise.

You might like to have a pen and paper to hand to take note of any insights that reveal themselves to you.

First, close your eyes and tune in to your body. Is there an area of discomfort that's been niggling at you (perhaps a pain, or an area of tension, for example)? Sit with this for a moment, allowing yourself to feel the discomfort, then gently ask it,

'What wisdom would you like to share with me today?'

And just be still and listen.

You might not be aware of anything at first – that's okay. It can take us a little while to tune in to our body's way of communicating and don't forget that there could be many different forms of communication: a feeling, an image, an emotion or perhaps even words.

Trust that, even if you're not consciously aware of any message, the fact you've asked and taken the time to listen has opened up a channel for communication.

After a few minutes, regardless of the outcome, thank your body for connecting with you and let it know that you intend to commit to this new dialogue over the coming weeks and months. Feel free to ask it to help you understand what it seeks to share with you. In time, you'll develop a closer relationship and supportive bond together.

Whatever you are keeping a note of from this and other exercises will form part of your 'reflective journal' which is the starting point to your W·I·L·D® journey. As we go through the various stages, your journal will grow.

And remember to play with everything I have suggested here. As children, we play all the time, yet as adults, we don't – but play is so important, whatever age we are. It helps to take us out of our stress system (the Sympathetic Nervous System) and into the relaxation system (the Parasympathetic Nervous System) because when we are playing, we are having fun.

Play is a great way to learn and is often more effective than just reading or following along. All of the exercises within this book are designed for you to play with and customise in any way that you find most effective. Don't be afraid to follow your discoveries wherever they may lead and approach them with a sense of fun. Not only will this move you into a more positive and relaxing mind space, but it will also help to free up your creativity, flexibility and problem-solving skills. There is no right or wrong!

Play, in my book, is definitely a win-win.

An important fact to note is something that I wasn't aware of when I first became poorly many years ago, though it seems obvious now.

When we are under stress, our digestive system isn't able to function properly.

We've all experienced feelings of nausea and perhaps lack of appetite at times of stress or anxiety - before a test or major life event, for example. Looking back now at the external stresses I was experiencing, it's no wonder that I developed food intolerances and a 'leaky' gut. When we are in the stress phase, we're too busy preparing for or actually engaging in 'fight or flight' to take the time needed to move into relaxation. Our entire body will then function in the stress phase continuously, and our gut is no exception to this.

If we marry this fact to the previous note regarding the messages our guts send to our brains, it becomes easy to see how our entire body is linked, even when two 'symptoms' or parts of our bodies may seem to have no logical relationship.

The Parasympathetic phase (which is our relaxation phase - also often referred to as our 'rest and digest' or 'rest and repair' phase) gives us a further clue about why it's so important to make time for relaxation in our lives. It is during this phase that our body digests what we've eaten and makes the resulting nutrients available to our cells so that they can undertake any maintenance, repair or healing work necessary.

Wonder, then, helps us to work with our bodies, discovering and exploring the things that make us feel relaxed and those which add to our stresses. Once we can really start to engage with these and experience the Wonder of our discoveries, then we can know how to support our bodies to enter that all-important parasympathetic state.

Before we leave Wonder, there's one last question you might like to explore:

- Consider: What takes you into 'The Zone' where you lose track of time, are lost in the moment and enjoy feelings of pure bliss?

If you can get into this 'zone,' I encourage you to access it as much as possible. The more time you can spend in feelings of bliss, the easier it will become to move forward on your wellness journey.

Chapter Summary

- We looked at living from the perspective of Wonder and learnt to open our minds and hearts to see the world through child-like eyes once more. This allows us to delight in the amazing creativity and abundance of the Universe.

- We learnt that, as humans, we are wired for a negative bias because it forms part of our survival strategy and keeps us alert for threats and danger; however, our 'core system' has not yet realised that we're living in a new millennium and no longer need to battle daily with predators. This results in our 'fight or flight' reactions flooding us with hormones which are not being utilised. They are left with nowhere to go and instead result in a sense of inner discomfort and unease.

- We understood that if we don't address this negative bias appropriately and safely, we can end up feeling exhausted, burnt out, frustrated and cynical. However, when we make a conscious effort to foster this child-like perspective of Wonder, we can start to appreciate the beauty and majesty of all things.

~ Six ~

W·I·L·D®
I is for Intuition

Inside Chapter Six

The 'I' of W·I·L·D® focuses on Intuition and how this supports our wellbeing. Here we'll be looking at:

• what this inner sense gives us
• why it's so important
• why and how we might feel we've lost touch with it
• and how we can take steps to reconnect with and strengthen it.

~ ~ ~ ~ ~

Did you know that our cells hold memory for us? In fact, before we developed language, this was one of the key ways in which our bodies remembered things and stored information for us. It explains why we can sometimes react strongly to something with a deep sense of discomfort or fear, even though we might not have any conscious memory of a trauma. Our cells just know it. This is Intuition. It is our inner sense of whether something is safe and/or a good fit for us.

Intuition (in-tuition) can be defined as an *'inner knowing, a guidance that we receive from our heart brain, our gut brain, and our body's wisdom'.*

When we lived as hunter-gatherers, this sense would have let us know when there was a predator nearby and whether or not it was on the hunt. If you watch wildlife programmes, you will see examples of predators, such as lions, walking through a herd of prey animals, like zebra or antelope. At times, the prey will not react. Their intuition will tell them that the hunter is not hungry and they are, therefore, safe. At other times, their intuition will tell them that the hunter is, in fact, seeking food and that they are in danger, so they will run. The difference between whether the hunter is hungry or not is something these prey animals just 'know'. It is the same for us humans. Think about those times when you've felt someone was watching you, and then, when you look up, you see their eyes on you. That's *your* intuition working.

At a base level, intuition is our safety mechanism. It alerts us to something that we may or may not need to respond to, which is why it is vital for us to tune in and pay attention to it. And why it is the second letter of W·I·L·D®.

Knowing how key our intuition is, it's important to be aware of two elements that must be in place in order to be able to hear, listen to and follow it:

• stillness
• authenticity (the attachment vs authenticity concept)

Two elements which can be challenging to find in our fast-paced noisy society.

Stillness (spaces of quiet) are hard to find when we are bombarded with news '24-7-365' via our computers and mobile devices. Our phones ping regularly throughout the day with updates and messages, all calling for our attention, so it does take a degree of commitment to set aside time for creating stillness for ourselves. However, embracing the power of profound inner stillness transforms us at the very core of our being. When we allow ourselves to rest deeply, the benefits unfold in beautiful ways: it recharges and refreshes us, acts as a powerful healer, and gently opens us up to the whispers of our inner guidance. This deep connection ensures we are moving in harmony with our true path, led by our inner wisdom.

If you feel ready to explore this, you might like to take a look at the Self-Care Exercise Playlist on my YouTube channel *(https://equenergy. com/SelfCareExercises)* and my Create Your Own W·I·L·D® Wellbeing programme, both of which share resources that can support you in this.

When we wish to access our intuition, we need to be in our True Nature, i.e. to be authentic. As infants, we have two basic needs - **Attachment** and **Authenticity** - but if these two are in conflict, i.e. if we sense that being authentic threatens our attachment, then it's the authenticity which will get sacrificed, for without attachment, we cannot survive. Yet, in my experience, authenticity is essential as it enables us to be true to ourselves and thus access the wisdom our body holds for us. This is our intuition. Let's explore this further.

Authenticity:

As infants, we might sense that our parent's attachment changes when we cry – for example they could become angry, frustrated or more distant. This may lead to us 'pushing down' our feelings and/or suppressing our natural emotions. We do this so that our parents will continue to care for us; however, in pushing down the feelings, we're cutting ourselves off from our inner knowledge of what is right for us as individuals – which puts us at risk of suppressing our Authenticity.

The fear of losing our parent's (caregiver's) love and care feels like a threat of death since our subconscious mind sees the world in 'black and white' and so recognises only two options - survival or death - with nothing in between. This means Attachment will always take precedence over Authenticity. In fact, to our subconscious mind, Authenticity can literally feel life-threatening because we may be going against our caregiver and, thus, could end up in danger.

This causes a problem. On one side, our rational brain may be telling us that we must not lose our attachment, however, our intuition might be uncomfortable at the loss of authenticity. These two opposing senses can, therefore, cause us to be confused which results in cognitive dissonance.

If this situation continues, we are in danger of growing up to be people-pleasers for whom being authentic feels alien, perhaps even scary. Is it any wonder, then, that some of us no longer know what our authentic self looks or feels like? And if we find ourselves wondering who our authentic self is, then we cannot fully access our intuition.

One of the most common ways in which we lose our authenticity is by buying into the stories society tells us about life. In her book 'Women Who Run with The Wolves,' Clarissa Pinkola Estes explores fairy tales and myths that are widely used to teach children about life. These fables originated in oral stories, which were told well before written records were created.

As Ms Estes writes in her introduction:

> "Stories are embedded with instructions which guide us about the complexities of life." [1]

Unfortunately, many of the old, original tales were latterly considered too dark for young ears and minds, and so they were 'softened', creating characters such as the Disney 'Fairy Godmother', or changed to conform to the beliefs and teachings of later generations. Ms Estes continues:

> "Sometimes various cultural overlays disarray the bones of stories … Over the course of time, old pagan symbols were overlaid with Christian ones, so that an old healer in a tale became an evil witch, a spirit became an angel … Sexual elements were omitted. Helping creatures and animals were often changed into demons and boogeys." [2]

Her conclusion is that the original teachings have become diluted or even lost. In fact, many of these tales have been altered to the point where they now teach completely different values, such as 'nice girls don't get angry' and that being 'sweet' will eventually win you the prince whom you'll marry and live 'happily ever after'.

---

1   *Women Who Run With The Wolves, Clarissa Pinkola Estes, p14*
2   *Women Who Run With The Wolves, Clarissa Pinkola Estes,*

Just think of Cinderella and all she put up with at the hands of her stepmother and the ugly sisters. The story – taken literally - seems to say that keeping quiet and accepting the bullying behaviour of others will ultimately pay off as the prince will come along to rescue the damsel, and she will live happily ever after. What a shock, then, as young girls, to find that real life doesn't actually work that way. Princes rarely come rushing to the rescue - and anyway, she's more than capable of rescuing herself! (Of course, these beliefs might not be held consciously, but they can still impact us on a subconscious level.)

Submitting to behaviours in others (that we find uncomfortable and even threatening) is *"actually decided when girls are very young, usually before five years of age"*, writes Ms Estes. *"They are taught to not see, and instead to 'make pretty' all manner of grotesquery's whether they are lovely or not... This early training to 'be nice' causes women to override their intuitions. In that sense, they are actually purposefully taught to submit to the predator."*

This makes it all the more difficult for us to trust our intuition. Our intuition might be shouting at us to do something differently, though this may be at odds with societal norms and teachings which strongly encourage us to 'quietly accept such behaviour and not make a fuss'.

In addition, although rationally we might know life isn't like a fairy tale, there's often still a part of us that believes if we do all the 'right' things, make all the 'right' choices and bend over backwards to please everyone around us, then things will work out, and we'll be happy. In reality, this is rarely – if ever – the case because it goes against our True Nature. **What we need to understand is that our True Nature is not about being a people pleaser, putting everyone else first and ourselves last, but about finding ways to express who we really are.** Once we discover this, it will allow us to live the life that we choose and show us what is right for us as an individual.

It might seem like I'm making a big issue of something that doesn't seem all that important; however, look at how little boys are raised to be outgoing, engage in rough and tumble and become adventurous, and contrast this with girls who are encouraged to be more thoughtful, caring and empathetic. The clothes on the shelves also reflect this, with the boys' aisles being dominated by bold primary colours, Batman and other superhero figures with slogans such as 'Kapow!', whereas the girls' aisles feature more pastel colours, soft and frilly clothes with statements like 'Daddy's Little Princess'. If you haven't been down the children's clothing aisles recently, then I recommend you take a look, and you'll see what I mean. **Note: I'm not saying that either of these is 'wrong', just that it creates stereotyping and subconscious expectations of behaviour.**

What, then, can we do if we've lost touch with our authenticity (maybe from childhood lessons as we navigate how to survive) and perhaps have learnt – in our subconscious cellular memory – that to be authentic threatens our safety? (Think back to the example of the child ceasing to cry to please its mother, even though to cry would be expressing its True Nature). How, then, do we reconnect with this ability and know what is right for us so that we can choose that above pleasing others?

Remember: thinking of ourselves is not necessarily selfish; often, it can be selfless. If an aeroplane is about to crash, you are instructed to put your own oxygen mask on before helping anyone else, not to save yourself alone and thus be selfish, but because you need to be able to breathe first so that you can help others. It is, therefore, a selfless act. If we look after ourselves first, then we can look after others in a more helpful and beneficial way.

Reconnecting with our Intuition

An exercise that can gently help us reconnect with both stillness and intuition is the Body Scan[3] I've previously mentioned. This scan will help us to quieten and focus our mind before tuning into the feelings and sensations of our body, assisting us in developing a personal 'body vocabulary' awareness. It might take some time and persistence, particularly if you are someone who has learnt that silence, emotions and authenticity are threatening, but try to persevere, and you will get there.

---

3   *https://equenergy.com/BodyScan/*

◆ Exercise: Tuning into your Inner Wisdom

Take a few moments now to pause and go through a Body Scan.

Simply observe and notice what feelings and sensations are coming up for you at this time, perhaps brought to the surface as you read this chapter. Make a note of any tension or discomfort. These are nudges from your Intuition, messages that your body is carrying something for you to explore, a wisdom to share to help you know yourself more fully and so be better equipped to support your wellbeing.

Sit with these feelings with curiosity and compassion if you can. Gently ask your body to reveal whatever is underlying these sensations, and then get still and see if anything comes to you.

You might get an answer straight away, or it might become clear over the coming days. If there doesn't seem to be anything, ask again or ask your body to help you understand. Let go of any expectations or attachment to getting an answer and simply allow it to become clear, trusting it will do so in just the right way and with perfect timing.

Conversely, you might struggle to connect with any feelings. As Gabor Maté says:

"There are two possibilities why your memories of childhood are so hazy... Either nothing happened worth remembering, or too much happened that may be hurtful for you to recall. ... human beings can tune out entire periods of their lives that were characterized by emotional pain."[4]

---

4 *Scattered Minds: The Origins and Healing of Attention Deficit Disorder, Gabor Maté*

The same can apply to our feelings today. If, during any of this process or exercises, you are beginning to uncover emotions and sensations that are either uncomfortable or confusing, then I would strongly advise reaching out for support. You may wish to consult a professional such as a counsellor or therapist. Alternatively, I would love you to reach out to me via email (robyn@equenergy.com) and let me know if you are concerned or struggling with this process. I am more than happy to offer any guidance I can and will work with you to find a suitable programme, if need be, that will most benefit you and your journey.

Alternatively I can highly recommend a book by Gemma Margerison entitled *'Connected: The 12 Ways of Wellbeing for a Holistically Healthy Life'*. It was published in 2021, during the Covid pandemic, when Gemma noticed that there were so many people in need of wellbeing support. In order to create this valuable resource, Gemma interviewed over 40 practitioners to create this book, which showcases the wide range of support options available. She has also categorised them into different aspects of wellbeing to assist the reader in their search. (You can find me in the chapter on Spiritual Wellbeing).

> **TIP:** If you're unsure about how to choose the practitioner that's right for you, I've written a blog post sharing my top tips on finding the best match: *7 Tips for Finding the Practitioner Who's Right For You* (link in the Resources at the end of the book).

What about the more challenging parts of this inner wisdom?

When engaging in the Body Scan, you might discover you're feeling emotions that you find uncomfortable – a common one is anger.

Many of us have learnt that anger is an 'unwanted', 'unhealthy' or maybe even 'dangerous' emotion. I know that as a child, I was afraid of anger in other people and also learnt that I was not supposed to show this myself as it wasn't a 'nice' emotion and 'good' girls didn't get angry. I didn't realise until much later that anger could be healthy and that there are appropriate ways to express it where no one needs to feel afraid or hurt.

I've also since learnt that anger is just another of our body's communication systems.

> ⭐ **TIP:** Think of anger as an internal 'intruder alarm', designed to let us know when one of our boundaries or values has been threatened or breached. In the same way that an intruder alarm in our homes can help us to feel safe, anger works to protect us. If we feel anger, it is generally a warning that we are not okay, so it's good to then explore why we are angry and address the root cause. We don't need to be afraid or ashamed of it, and we don't need to push it down or suppress it; it's about recognising its origins so that we can find a more healthy and safe way to express it.

Also, suppressing our anger can have a detrimental effect. Keeping it 'bottled up' and not finding a (healthy) way to release it can negatively impact our energy. Not only that, but we tend to experience a loss of clarity when we don't explore and address our anger, which means the boundaries we have worked so hard to put in place can be compromised. If we continue to believe that anger (or any other 'negative' emotion) is 'wrong', then experiencing these feelings will push us into a 'fight or flight' response, which in turn chips away at our connection with our True Nature. Remember, we need stillness and calm to really connect with our true selves, and harbouring uncomfortable energy will have the opposite effect.

We may work diligently to discover our sense of Self, but then, if we become overwhelmed with anger (or other uncomfortable emotions), we might seek to disconnect from this discomfort, but this actually results in us disconnecting from our intuitive knowing of what is/is not supportive for us. Effectively we've stopped listening to our intuition. And so, begins a vicious circle.

When this happens, and we enter this vicious circle, the separation between 'Self' and 'Other' can become blurred, and we can lose sight of who we are.

For simplicity: 'Self' in this sense refers to things we can control, and 'Other' refers to things we cannot. For example, how another person reacts to a situation or what their belief system is falls under the umbrella of 'other'. We cannot control these in the same way we cannot control certain elements of our environment, such as the layout of a supermarket. When we have our own thoughts, which are independent of others, these become what is known as our 'Self'. 'Self' includes environmental elements that we can control (think about the safe place we discussed previously), as well as our thoughts, values and beliefs.

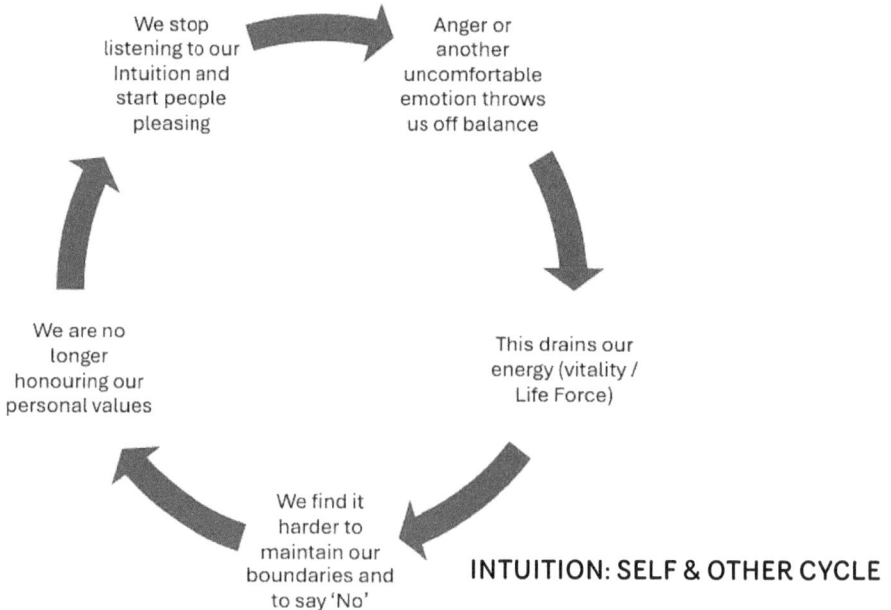

We stop listening to our Intuition and start people pleasing

Anger or another uncomfortable emotion throws us off balance

This drains our energy (vitality / Life Force)

We are no longer honouring our personal values

We find it harder to maintain our boundaries and to say 'No'

INTUITION: SELF & OTHER CYCLE

Hence, our sense of 'Self' supports our intuition. Your thoughts, values, beliefs, emotions, etc – all the things that make you You and that are within your control - connect you to your own personal wisdom. It's a bit like tuning a radio dial to our own inner frequency. Your 'True Nature' channel. From 'Self' and with the support of intuition, we can become clearer on how to make choices and follow paths which will ultimately prove beneficial to our wellbeing. If we are open to our intuition, we will be able to hear our 'Self' providing guidance and pushing us in the direction of learning and growth.

If we don't listen to ourselves and instead take on the noise (thoughts) of 'Other' and ignore emotions such as anger, then the signal from our True Nature channel can be drowned out, making it harder to connect with our 'Self' guidance.

I appreciate this can be a difficult concept to get your head around; the main thing to remember here is that we should embrace our emotions in a way which supports the most favourable outcome for ourselves, regardless of external factors. If you are unsure how to make this work for you, I encourage you to reach out for support from a professional. If we've lost a sense of the boundaries between our 'Self' and 'Other', this will also impact on our wellbeing as our body is no longer clear on what is 'me' and what is 'not me'. It no longer knows what to 'keep out' and what is 'safe', so these two become confused. Studies have shown that suppressing our emotions contributes to conditions classed as 'autoimmune diseases'[5] where the body is said to be 'attacking itself'. In fact, its systems are in overdrive in an attempt to survive.

We can conclude, therefore, that allowing ourselves to tune into our bodies and listen to our emotions is good for our wellbeing. It will help us to get clear on how we feel about things, remind us of what our values are, and denote where we wish to draw our boundaries. This level of connection to our body will also open us up to the wisdom it holds and seeks to share with us, and the more we practice this, the more our intuition will speak to us. Thus, the stronger and clearer its voice will become.

Exercise: Identify Your Values

To discover your own unique set of values, I recommend pausing here and trying the following exercise.

- Turn to Appendix 4 and take a look at the list of values given there.

- Go through the list to see which ones resonate with you. You'll probably end up with quite a long list!

- Narrow the list down to your top ten and then your top three.

- This will help you identify your values. You can then consider these when making choices and deciding which options are best for you.

---

5   https://www.youtube.com/watch?v=KSc1GDNC4b4

- Getting clear on your values can also help you understand why things feel 'good' to you or why they feel 'off', which in turn will make it easier for you to explain your perspective to others.

Exploring our connection in this way will also help us to recognise the various 'voices' that make up our inner guidance: our 'head voice', 'gut voice' and 'heart voice'.

It's worth noting that when I say 'voice', your intuition and its teachings might not come to you as words. When we ask questions of it, our 'voice' can 'speak' to us in various ways:

- In something we read.
- In something we hear.
- The lyrics of a song.
- A picture that we see.
- A feeling or 'sense'.
- An inner image that feels like a confirmation or 'knowing' in answer to an issue you've been pondering.

So don't worry if you aren't getting words. Your unique inner voice might just be seeking to communicate in a different way, and that's okay. Just be open to this and 'listen'—pay attention—with all of your senses.

Now, when I am practising, I listen to each voice in turn and find the best balance between them to guide me. You will come to recognise each of your voices like this:

- Our *head-brain* seeks to rationalise and be logical but can get caught up in 'analysis paralysis' – overthinking.
- Our *heart-brains* are loving and passionate but are not particularly practical.
- Our *gut-brain* focuses on how things feel and can give us a sense of whether or not our plans and values are a good fit for us. The gut-brain, though, can sometimes get lost down emotion-filled rabbit holes.

If you take the three together, it becomes like our own inner advisory committee where we can listen to each voice in turn and allow them to balance each other out. The response from our gut-brain, for example, may benefit from the rationalisation of our head-brain. It can take time to achieve this level of clarity, but once we have, then it's simply a case of listening to each argument, evaluating their strengths and weaknesses and choosing the course of action we feel is most appropriate.

Practical example (to assist with your understanding of this exercise):

When my husband and I were thinking about moving to Wales, it felt like a huge decision, and I had so many questions. I'd never lived in the countryside before. Would I like it? Would I be able to cope with the different pace of life and being in a much more remote location? It was the perfect opportunity to listen to the wisdom from my head, my heart and my gut. My head looked at the practicalities of what living in a rural location would be like and all the physical changes this would bring to our lives and routines. My heart considered my desire to be closer to Nature and how important this was to me, compared with the advantages of living in Bristol. My gut tuned in to what was right for me and what would best support my wellbeing. There were advantages and disadvantages to both options but exploring them from these different perspectives helped me to reach a truly informed decision.

Of course, there were still aspects of this new life that I could not have foreseen, but getting as clear as I could possibly be on why I had made this particular choice, I was able to navigate issues with a greater sense of clarity and direction.

How to know that your intuition is speaking to you

You might feel drawn to taking a different route on a regular journey or discover a new road that is pulling you to explore. Whilst this may feel like a whim, you may find that if you listen to that voice and take the alternative route or explore the new road, it will result in a positive outcome. You might, for example, drive past a banner advertising a show at the weekend that you'd love to attend.

Sometimes, we will suddenly think of an old friend or acquaintance that we haven't seen in a long time. Later that day, they might phone you out of the blue to share some exciting news. Similarly, if you get a feeling that you should call a particular person, that is also our intuition working and telling us that we need to check in on that individual.

You might begin to see a particular number repeatedly on clocks, number plates, buses, and so on; then, when you look up the meaning, you discover that it's a message with particular significance for you[6].

These are all prime examples of our intuition giving us a little nudge, so it can be good to practice noticing these nudges and maybe even write them down. You might start to spot patterns or even just become aware of how often this actually happens.

The more you pay attention, the more frequently your intuition will 'speak' to you.

In the next few pages, we will explore some specific exercises that can help you to really connect with and listen to your intuition.

◆ Exercise: Intuitive 'Nudges'

Thinking back to those little 'nudges' we get from our intuition, I invite you to play with this idea.

- Start by taking some time to yourself so that you can reflect on your day and any nudges you may have encountered.
- Make a note of these and then start to pay them some attention.
- Play with the ideas and messages you are discovering and know that you can't get it 'wrong'. It isn't a 'test', and you can't 'fail'. All you need to do is pay attention to those inner prompts.

---

6 *If you would like to explore this further, take a look at the book 'Spirology Reflection of Self - The Road Back to Me' by Amanda Bowden.*

- Then, explore the prompts and respond. Take a different route, for example, or spot the times when you are thinking of someone and they come to you in a certain way—perhaps they will call you or you will receive a card, letter, or email.
- Notice repeating patterns and explore what these might mean for you. This exercise is a great way to develop your intuitive 'muscle' and tune in to its frequency.

Other ways you can listen to your intuition

Another way to listen to your intuition is to notice your dreams. They can offer us wisdom, though it's often shared in a metaphorical rather than a literal sense. For example, I used to dream of tornados when I felt that my life was 'spiralling out of my control'. Keeping a pen and some paper by your bed will allow you to write down as much of your dream as you can remember as soon as you wake. Keeping a record will help you spot any recurring themes and where the dreams (potentially) relate to events in your waking life. When you take notice of these dreams, your intuition will also receive the subconscious message that you are open to receiving its messages in this way.

You can also explore:

- drawing power cards and seeing how often their message is an answer to an inner question you've been asking – or ask a specific question and see what card(s) you draw. There are many different kinds of power cards available, so choose the one(s) that you feel drawn to. I have several packs that I've picked up along the way that either relate to personal interests (my Colour pack) or that have been made by people or groups I've connected with (such as my White Lion pack, my horse pack and my Self-Love Creativity pack).

- muscle testing to connect directly with your body's wisdom. Our muscles hold memory and respond from our body's blueprint which knows exactly what it needs in order to function at its optimum (at any given time). We can, therefore, tap into this knowledge in order to find answers to our questions. Muscle testing can be accessed in various different ways. I often use a sway test or pendulum.

◆ Exercise: The Sway Test

- To do a sway test, start by standing up straight with your feet about hip distance apart and knees soft. (**Health & Safety note: Make sure you keep your eyes open and you have plenty of space before engaging in this exercise.**)

- Next, you need to 'calibrate' your sway, which means learning how your body sways depending on the validity of the statement you are making. To do this, say a phrase such as 'My name is Rumpelstiltskin' and notice which way your body sways. Assuming your name isn't actually Rumpelstiltskin (!), this direction will be your 'no', i.e. the way your body will sway if a negative response is being given.

- Next, repeat the exercise, this time saying 'My name is…' using your real name - the one that feels true to you (this could be a nickname or either the full or a shortened form of your given name) and again see which way you sway. This direction becomes your 'yes'. (I normally sway forwards for 'yes' and backwards for 'no', but you might be the other way around, or you might even sway from side to side rather than forwards and backwards).

- If you find that you're not swaying, it could be because you're dehydrated, so try taking a drink of water (not fizzy drinks, fruit juice, coffee, tea or even herbal tea, but plain water). You could also be a bit 'dysregulated', so you can try the 'Cook's Hook Up' exercise in Appendix 3 to help you re-regulate before trying again.

- Once you have calibrated your sway, you can create a series of statements to use with this test in order to help get to the understanding that you're looking for. Remember you need to use statements where you're looking for a 'yes' / 'no' response only.

◆ Further Intuition Development Exercises:

1. Pendulum dowsing[7]. I learned how to dowse with a pendulum a few years ago. It's a very simple skill to develop once you get started, though if this is new for you, it can be good to find someone who can help you. Once you get going, it's a similar process to the sway test above, using statements and seeing whether you get a 'yes' or 'no' movement from the pendulum.

2. Use a pack of playing cards and lay them face down. Using only your intuition, see if you can guess the colour/suit/value of the card at the top of the pile, or even whether the card is of a high or low value, a number or a picture card. See how many times your intuition is right.

3. Get a set of colour swatch cards, such as paint sample cards, and place them face down. Then, without looking, see if you can get a sense of the colour – is it dark or light? Does it bring up any other sensations? Can you guess the colour even?

4. Buy or make a set of cards with simple drawings on them, such as a square, a triangle, a circle, a book, or a table. Place these face down and pull one out at random. Without looking at the picture, see if you can get a sense of what it might be and then draw it onto a piece of paper. Alternatively, you can ask a partner to draw something that you can't see and then you try to draw what you think is on their paper.

5. Practising the *Hakalau*. One meaning of Hakalau is *"To stare at, as in meditation and to allow to spread out."* If you've never tried it before, it can be incredibly powerful though it may take a few attempts to master it.

   • To begin, stare at a spot that's just above eye level – so that your eyes feel like they're 'bumping off' your eyebrows.

   • Look at this spot until it goes fuzzy, a ring appears around it, or it appears to move.

   ---
   7   *'Pendulum dowsing is a form of divination that uses a weighted object usually a crystal or gemstone hung from a metal chain or pendant to tap into your intuition for spiritual guidance'.* www. sunrisedirect.co.uk

- When this happens, look away, then stare at the spot again.

- Now allow your focus to soften and open out so that you become aware of your peripheral vision as well as what's directly in front of you. (You can find a full description of the exercise in Appendix 5.)

- Practising the Hakalau helps to still and open your mind, making you more receptive to the nudges of your intuition

6. Listen to guided meditations. Often, within these meditations, you are encouraged to visualise objects, people or places, so spending time each day meditating can be a really great way to develop your visualisation skills. What you then specifically visualise in relation to the meditation prompts is the result of your subconscious working and connecting with your inner being. Making a note of these can improve your self-awareness and increase your understanding of your intuition. Guided meditations are readily available online, but if you are not sure where to begin, then take a look at those on my website at *www.equenergy.com/meditations*.

7. Vision boarding (literally creating a 'board' of pictures) can be another great way to develop your intuition. When you have an image of what you'd like to achieve, find things that reflect or represent this for you and put them together on your board. This can include pictures, words, photos, fabrics, textures, or anything that works for you. I've created 'future' bank statements and diary pages for my vision board. If you're manifesting your dream trip, for example, you might include an itinerary and create some 'travel tickets' for example, to make the vision feel more 'real' for you. Whilst it is preferable to create a physical board that you place somewhere visible, there are online resources you can use to create one, too.

All of these exercises are fun tools for you to experiment with; the most important thing is to observe and notice what comes up for you when you are trying any of them.

We're all different, so your discoveries will be unique to you.

For some people, their intuition is like an inner voice, for others, it's a feeling, whilst many more will see images in their mind's eye. There isn't a 'right' way to receive your intuition; it's about finding what works for you.

Why is intuition so important?

We can use our intuition to help us create the life that we want to live. As we tune into our body and ask for its guidance, we will develop our understanding of its vocabulary and build up a shared dialogue. Then, we can begin to hone our ability to listen and respond appropriately. Once we become more proficient, we can use these skills to help us make choices that will ultimately enrich our lives. Tools like the sway test, for example, can be incredibly helpful when it comes to those choices. Remember to use 'yes / no' statements, though, and use these to help you identify the next steps that best serve you or that will bring you closer to your goal.

Note: Believing in or relying on the tools we have discussed can be a huge leap of faith and may well be uncomfortable. You might receive a different response from the sway test, for example, than you were expecting, and that's okay. It is simply our body communicating from within rather than from our logical head-brain, but it is important to only follow the responses which feel right for you at the time. Learning to listen to and take note of our intuition is a process and requires a level of trust within ourselves that we may yet have to achieve. Start with small steps and choices and become comfortable with each before moving on and building up gradually to the big decisions.

Intuition and its relationship with Manifestation

It is difficult to talk about intuition in the way we're doing here without also considering its links to the practice of manifestation. For simplicity, manifesting can be defined as *'the practice of thinking aspirational thoughts with the purpose of making them real'*[8].

8   https://www.vox.com/the-goods/21524975/manifesting-does-it-really-work-meme

As we've already discussed, intuition will give us 'nudges', which are, in essence, the beginning of our journey towards the outcome we are aiming for. These nudges form messages which point us in the right direction and effectively function as our inner 'satnav' directing us towards the appropriate path. It is widely accepted that simply 'asking' the universe for guidance or an intended outcome and then sitting back and waiting for it to happen rarely achieves the results we desire.

However, that doesn't mean the universe isn't listening; it is simply that we are not listening to the messages it is sending in return – which are being delivered by our intuition. These communications will guide us towards certain actions, for example, that can ultimately end in a realisation of our original intention. Thus, it is virtually impossible for manifestation to work effectively without also understanding and listening to our intuition.

> **TIP:** When seeking to manifest something, the secret is to be able to 'experience' it, even before it's really there in your life. To do this you need to put your attention on the experience you wish to have, rather than on the wanting of it, or on thinking of what you don't want. This is a technique top athletes use in their training to help them excel. The Universe is very literal - if you think about wanting, you'll probably end up getting more wanting! (*Additional sources https://trueselfmanifestation.com/intuition-manifesting*)

Also, it doesn't understand negation, so if you focus on the thing you don't want, you'll get that and not your desired outcome. If it hears you focusing on something, it will simply see you spending a lot of time thinking about that thing so, to its way of reasoning, you must want it – and so it brings you more of it, even if you've been focusing on the thing you don't want! Thus, when we spend time focusing on how little money we have or how tired we feel, guess what – we continue to lack money and our tiredness increases.

If, instead, we could hold an image of ourselves living a life of abundance with all the energy we could possibly need, and if we are focusing on all the things we would love to do, then that is what the Universe will hear and, thus, deliver.

Further, the more time we spend thinking about something, the more we vibrate with that energy and attract similar energies into our experience – like a magnet. The more we can bring those higher vibrations of Joy, Gratitude and Wonder into our manifestations, the more we can imagine what our goal would look like, sound like, feel like, smell like and taste like. This leads to us becoming more closely matched with our desired outcome, which projects a stronger magnetic draw to the Universe.

Now that we've explored our intuition, hopefully, you can start to see it's all about relaxing into the process and trusting that 'this, or something even better' is, even now, on its way to us!

Chapter Summary

- We looked at various tools and exercises we could use in order to listen to our Intuition.

- We understood that this is about tuning in to our body and letting our inner wisdom speak to us.

- We learned how our intuition speaks to us through our emotions and physical sensations, and the more we listen, the more we will come to understand its particular vocabulary and language.

- We discovered that doing this (regularly) will help us to make decisions and take actions that are in alignment with our True Nature. Once we are in alignment with our True Nature, we can start to feel 'at home' in our skin and become the wonderful people we were born to be.

~ Seven ~

W·I·L·D®
L is for Loving (ourselves)
As we are and as we are not

Inside Chapter Seven

The 'L' of W·I·L·D® is all about learning to Love ourselves, just as we are, 'warts and all'. You are 'perfectly imperfect', and that is enough—you are enough. It's time to set aside trying and striving for perfection that does not exist and instead practice simply be-ing you.

~ ~ ~ ~ ~

Often, we are our own worst critic. We say things to ourselves that we would never say, even to our worst enemy. But why is this? Why do we beat ourselves up rather than cheer ourselves on?

There is actually a good reason. It's another one of those survival strategies that once served a purpose.

As we've touched on in the previous chapters, our inner voice has been working hard to keep us in line so that our caregivers will continue to provide us with the things we need. This means that, at one time, our inner voice was our best friend. It made sure we didn't lose the care we needed to survive, **but the problem is, this 'friend' (this little inner voice) doesn't grow up. It doesn't realise that we're now an adult, so it's like having a 4-year-old as your co-pilot or navigator, telling you where to go and how to drive.**

Dr Gabor Maté likens this to having what he calls a 'stupid friend':

> "…it came along as a protective thing. So rather than seeing it as negative, I encourage you to look at these characteristics as what we call stupid friends. They're friends because they came along to protect you. And the fear of commitment came along to protect you. The stupidity is that it doesn't learn that it's no longer needed. It can give you the same message, even though we are no longer this small child. And even though you have more capabilities. But they're friends. They don't come along to hurt you. They come along to help you."[1]

Added to this, our brains are wired intentionally with a negative bias, so we can pick up on anything that could pose a threat to our safety. These negativities are then retained in a file of memories telling us what is safe and what is not. When we come across something new, something that our brain doesn't recognise, the negative bias will mark this as potentially dangerous until it can be proven otherwise.

Over time, if we learn that our world is, on balance, a generally safe place, this alert system does dial down, but if experience has taught us that the world is scary, unpredictable and can potentially hurt or frighten us, then the dial will be turned right up, leaving us hypervigilant and jumpy. And this is when our inner voice is most likely to be activated. At this point, its purpose is to keep us safe, so it will respond by employing all manner of internal dialogue. This dialogue might tell us that we are stupid/not good enough/not brave enough, and because we are so used to this voice, we will take its comments on board. This can then lead us to retreat into our shell, 'armour up' or 'puff up' - whichever strategy we have learnt to keep ourselves safe.

If we take a step back to look at the effects of what we tell ourselves rather than the words we say, we can get a sense of what this inner voice is trying to achieve. Our adult self might not be happy with our

1   Trauma is a 'stupid friend' that our minds & bodies don't forget: Dr. Gabor Maté - CBC Podcasts
-        https://www.cbc.ca/radio/podcastnews/trauma-is-a-stupid-friend-that-our-minds-bodies-don-t-forget-dr-gabor-mat%C3%A9-1.6612920

behaviour, but our inner child might be celebrating that we've *survived another scary situation*.

To illustrate, my inner voice would regularly tell me that nobody would be interested in anything I had to say. There were times in my childhood when I'd felt ignored, overlooked or dismissed, which was painful and embarrassing for me, and I realise now that my inner voice (even in adulthood) was simply trying to save me from further feelings of shame by convincing me to stay quiet. Unfortunately, the outcome of this was that staying quiet (as an adult) left me feeling frustrated and annoyed with myself for being such a 'doormat' and allowing others to walk all over me.

When we hear our inner voice talking to us in a way that leaves us feeling 'negative' or 'less', we have to learn how to quieten it and show it how to be more supportive rather than critical and shaming. In short, we need to learn to Love ourselves. But how?

◆ Exercise: Dialogue with your Inner Self

Start by setting aside some time to ask these questions of your inner self. Afterwards, it's a good idea to have something fun planned to lift your mood and celebrate the action you have taken.

Thinking about your inner voice:

- How does it speak to you?
- What tone does it use?
- What words or phrases do you hear?
- Is it always words, or is it also feelings?
- Is it reflected in your body language?
- What sort of things does it say to you?
- When does it speak to you/when is it loudest?
- Are there particular people/situations that make it louder/more frequent/more critical/angry/shaming?
- Are there particular people/situations where it becomes gentler/softer/quieter?
- Do you recognise the tone/words/phrases?
- Have you heard these before, perhaps from a parent/caregiver/teacher?
- How does it make you feel?

You might like to journal on this to help you spot any patterns.

TIP/LIGHTBULB MOMENT: When you have a clearer sense of your inner critic, you'll probably notice that it's not actually yours at all! Often, you can start to break down your inner voice and pinpoint where some of its messages come/came from. At school, teachers might have told you that you were lazy and that you didn't try hard enough. If you carry this into adulthood, your inner voice will repeat that message, yet it's not a fact. It is messaging from others and not your own inner voice at all. In fact, your True Nature loves you - totally, unconditionally and without judgement, and it would never speak to you other than with absolute love and acceptance of you, exactly as you are.

This sounds incredibly confusing, so let's dig deeper. Where has this voice come from, and why does it (often) hold negative messages?

Essentially, our inner voice is comprised of a combination of messages we have heard over the years. These messages originated from others; however, we have internalised and identified with them, so they become ingrained as part of our inner voice. Because we are negatively wired, it is natural for us to remember the critical comments and repeat these to ourselves more readily than the positive ones.

Several studies around positive and negative messaging (including work by John Gottman and Robert Levenson, who closely studied the effects of negativity within couples) cite the 'magic ratio' of 5:1. The 'magic ratio' states that *'in order to overcome our negative bias, for every one negative encounter, we need to experience five positive encounters'*.

But if all of us have this negative bias, then it's understandable that our negative thoughts and comments will feature highly, not just in conversation with our inner voice but also in our external communications. In fact, this can easily become our habit and our norm. Think about how we Brits like to moan—especially about the weather!

When you start to notice that parts of this inner voice aren't yours, then you can take a step back and view it more objectively. You can see your voice as a character almost and understand that you have a choice to either listen to it or ignore it. Once we are able to see our inner voice in this way, we can separate it from ourselves and engage (with) it in unbiased dialogue.

Remember, this inner voice started out as our friend who wanted to keep us safe as a child, so rather than listening to its negative bias, we can instead thank it for its efforts over the years but let it know that it can stand down a little. We have matured enough to be in charge of our own safety.

We've got this now!

We can then choose when to let our inner voice share its concerns with us and, at the same time, pay attention to the emotion within the words and the tone it uses. This means not automatically taking on board its fears but rather looking for the unmet need which is hiding behind what it's saying. Because the 'unmet need' is what we need to address and resolve, then we will be well on the way to loving ourselves 'just as we are' (think Bridget Jones).

<u>How, then, do we identify this unmet need?</u>

The easiest way to do this is by creating that safe space we referenced in Chapter 3. Here, we can listen to our inner voice and feelings, and we can ask it questions with understanding and compassion. Take time here to listen to what your inner child is saying. *Note: You will need to do this more than once. Making it a regular habit can be beneficial.* Ask: How does it make you feel? What is the emotion? (If you are struggling to identify the emotion, the Emotion Wheel in Appendix 6 may be helpful).

> **TIP:** Remember, emotions are different to perceptions. A perception is an interpretation, the meaning that we put onto events, which is is coloured by our beliefs. Our perceptions might be true but on the other hand, they might not. They could easily be skewed by our fears.
>
> An *emotion*, however, just is. It is how we feel. It isn't right or wrong, it's just fact.

When we can name the emotion[2] we can then explore the need behind it. It could be, for example, that the need behind the emotion we identify is the need for acceptance or to be seen or feel safe.

When we have identified this need, then we can take steps to address

---

2   *Sometimes we can struggle to put a name to how we're feeling, particularly if we've been burying our emotions and haven't yet developed a vocabulary for them. If you're finding it difficult to put your emotions into words you could try using an Emotion Wheel – there are many examples available which are easily found in a Google search – or Emotion Cards. Personally, I use* **The Mood Cards: Make Sense of Your Moods and Emotions for Clarity, Confidence and Wellbeing** *from Anrea Harrn, which I bought on Amazon.*

it in more appropriate and healthy ways – remembering to bring in gentle, non-judgmental, compassionate curiosity which will help to shift our inner voice towards being more supportive and uplifting in its messaging and ultimately enabling us to love ourselves more deeply.

Addressing our unmet needs

If we have identified our unmet need as a lack of safety, for example, next, we can explore how we might bring in more of what helps us to feel safe. This could be talking to a particular friend, visiting a certain place, meditating, taking some time out ..., or whatever we feel would help us to feel calm and safe and, therefore, address that need.

Similarly, we might feel that we're not being truly seen/heard/understood/respected, so we can seek ways to address these needs too. Below, you'll find a few suggestions for how you can do this.

Remember that unmet needs are perfectly healthy, and it's both normal and natural to seek ways to meet them. When we gain awareness of what these needs are, we can find ways to support ourselves that feel empowering and liberating rather than coming from a place of fear and/or feelings of inferiority.

If you're finding it difficult to work out how to address or resolve these unmet needs, then I often find using the internet really helpful. You could search for something along the lines of, 'how can I earn greater respect' or 'how do I become a more effective communicator' etc... you get the idea. There are hundreds of resources out there, so it's just a case of narrowing them down to ones that are achievable and feel right for you.

Suggestions for addressing unmet needs:

1. Take time to breathe and listen to your body.
   - This helps us to get centred and calm and to have greater clarity so that we can share our thoughts more effectively.

2. Engage in self-care – showing ourselves that we are deserving of respect and that we are worth listening to.

3. Learn some assertiveness techniques to hone our listening and sharing skills.
   - I used to think that no one listened to me, that they didn't want to hear what I had to say, but later, I realised that I wasn't speaking from a place of assurance and clarity, and that was why no one listened. Think confident salesman vs nervous salesman. Both have the same message, but the confident salesman will deliver it with assurance and is therefore listened to over the one who is nervous.

4. Notice the things our inner voice says that make us feel uncomfortable in some way – for example, shame, guilt or hurt. We can then try to reframe these thoughts and create a narrative that feels more uplifting and supportive.

In the example above, where I felt no one listened to me, I explored new thoughts I could create that would help me feel a little bit better and decided to teach my inner voice some new phrases.

For example:

√ I listen to and respect myself.
√ I have value to share.
√ I share my thoughts in a clear and respectful way, and people listen to my point of view.
√ I listen to other people's perspectives, and together, we find a way that works for us both.

When you are re-educating your inner voice, you need to teach it something you believe so that you can really embed the new thoughts and not just dismiss them. Our ultimate goal - to experience happiness, joy and inner calm – might be too big a leap at first, but every step in that direction is a 'win'.

In our society, we can often feel that we're judged for our 'performance'

– think of all the exams, tests and assessments you've had to do throughout your life. I know that, for me, I often felt the focus was more on what I could remember and repeat rather than on what I thought or who I was as a person. I grew up believing there was one right answer, and if I didn't give that, then I'd failed.

In some situations, this may be true, but in much of life, this isn't the case. However, if our default is to believe we have failed and given the 'wrong answer', it can leave us feeling we're not good enough, which then erodes any trust we have in our own thoughts and abilities. This will then (in our minds) add further credence to the negative messages our inner voice is sending, which means we are at risk of not listening to any of its positive messages.

It's the same with intelligence. Our benchmarks for intelligence are often based on a particular set of 'norms' which don't make allowance for other ways of looking at/experiencing/interacting with the world. The risk here is that if we are judging everyone by the same metrics, we may 'sideline' those whose norms are different to these idealistic benchmarks. I think this is a huge loss to society. The benchmarks are based on historical methods of measurement, which are not as relevant today as they once were. Just because someone doesn't meet or match these criteria doesn't mean they don't have an equal value to those who do. Only by embracing all of our differences can we truly experience the wonderful variety, colour and flavour of life, which add to the richness of our culture and society. We need to be able to see things in new ways in order to create, develop and ultimately grow.

Let me share an example:

My first career was as a Sign Language interpreter. The people I worked with were labelled as 'deaf and dumb' and were often dismissed. The word 'dumb', in particular, has evolved in meaning over the years, and rather than simply referencing a person without speech, it is now more commonly used to suggest a person of lower intelligence. People have varying levels of intelligence, and this is true whether or not they are members of the Deaf community, so when the word 'dumb' is used nowadays, it can be deemed highly offensive. Just because people are unable to hear or use a spoken language, it doesn't automatically mean they are of a lower intelligence. Let's not forget that the Deaf community uses a visual language which is beautiful, complex and highly expressive and if we ignore this or consider them to be dumb and marginalise them (or any other community), we won't embrace the rich wonder and variety of our world.

It is not okay to be closed-minded and sideline those who might not fit the generalised societal 'norms'. Not only is this offensive, rude and disrespectful, we are ignoring all that they have to offer. Deaf people, for example, are highly visual and have much to share in regard to the concepts of 'space' and 'place'. Also, people with neurodiversity might view the world from a slightly different perspective and, therefore, be able to offer insights that others will have missed.

These are simple examples from my work and life, but I am sure you can think of many more. In short, having a different perspective adds to – rather than detracts from – the richness of society as a whole.

But, often, society misses out on the wonderful gifts **everyone** can bring because we don't understand or feel able to be open to the beauty of our differences.

Loving ourselves against society's expectations

Society happily judges us on surface appearances – how we look. We're bombarded daily through social media, television, billboards, magazines, etc., with images of what someone or a select group of people has decided is 'beautiful' and what we should, therefore, look like. At the moment, for women, this is generally slim, often pale-skinned, young and with long blonde hair. For men, it's having lots of muscular definition, and in many circles, you might find only these two gender types shown.

Where, then, do you fit in if you don't look this way? If you're taller/shorter/larger/smaller/red-haired/use a wheelchair/are an amputee/learn in a different way/identify with a different gender/are blind/deaf … the list goes on.

Society is slowly starting to embrace these differences, changing the 'norm' and moving away from the stereotypes, but magazine covers and advertisements (to name just two) still typically revert to that 'beautiful' ideal, which is impossible for most of us to achieve. With this external and societal focus on appearance, our inner voice is given more than enough fodder to continue criticising us for how we look, which takes us into a negative spiral. In addition, not only will it tell us that we don't meet the 'norm', but it could also take on the blaming and shaming which so often accompanies these media messages.

> **TIP:** When we read something, we 'hear' it internally. This means we can receive the message with double the impact - seeing it in print and hearing it internally. The result of our inner voice listening to these outside messages is not good. It is all too common to experience a disconnection from, a lack of love for, and even a mistrust of, this body in which we live. This, exacerbated by external commentary, can lead to a deep discomfort within our own skin.

If you remember my story at the beginning, I certainly felt this way. For me, it began when I was a teenager and a doctor commented on my size, inferring that I was overweight. Up until that point, I'd only really thought about my body in terms of what it allowed me to do – walk, ride my bike, swim, eat, sleep, and generally go about my day-to-day life, but suddenly I became conscious of how I looked and what others thought of me. It wasn't long before I was on a downhill spiral in my relationship with my body.

That particular doctor was someone I was seeing because of an issue with my knees. I had a condition which isn't uncommon in childhood, but most people grow out of it by their teens. I hadn't, so I was having further tests and treatment. I genuinely believed that there was something 'wrong' with my knees, and when the treatment failed, I started to blame my weight for causing these issues simply because the doctor suggested this could be a contributing factor.

As I revealed at the start of this book, my parents separated when I was thirteen, which was incredibly stressful. Whilst I was undergoing all of these medical tests and treatment for my knees, professionals focused on my weight and what was happening to my kneecaps, but not one person asked if I was okay or what was going on at home. Now I realise the difference it could have made if they had opened up this dialogue.

What was going on at home was a major contributing factor to my health issues, and perhaps, had this been raised, I might have been able to develop a better relationship with my body and avoid some of the problems I later experienced.

Through my wellness journey, I have learnt that symptoms are signals from our body which give us vital information about what is and isn't working in our lives. If we are able to listen and unpack those signals, we can discover everything we need to know. We can learn, for example, why the symptom appeared at this particular time, in this particular part of our body, and in that particular way. The knowledge we gain from taking the time to listen gives us the insight we need to support ourselves and head back to wellbeing again.

I realise now that my knees weren't going wrong at all; my body wasn't making a mistake, attacking itself or letting me down; it was just trying to tell me that there was an issue I needed to address. If I'd known how to listen back then, I would have also understood the issue, but sadly, I wouldn't learn how to hear and interpret my body's language until many years later. This is the power of loving vs not-loving ourselves.

When I was going through these issues and believing that my knees were 'going wrong', my relationship with my body became increasingly unhealthy. My negative bias caused me to focus on the 'problem' and my associated fears: Will my knees ever get better? Will I be in worsening pain for the rest of my life? - which only exacerbated the issue that had created the symptoms in the first place. It was a vicious cycle.

◆ Exercise: Somatic Journaling

I encourage you to pause here and return to the somatic journaling exercise I shared on page 123. This is a great way to practice exploring the symptoms and signals our body is sending and identifying any unhelpful messaging that we can reverse as we continue our journey towards wholehearted love.

As humans, we have a well-developed cerebral cortex[3] that allows us to view the world from a metaphorical perspective as much as from a literal one. This, we now know, is reflected in how the tissues of our body react to emotional stresses.

☆ **DID YOU KNOW?**

Many of the symptoms we experience in our muscular-skeletal system relate to our sense of self-worth just as much as our ability and strength to do things.

If we take our basic skeleton as an example, we can see that its role is to provide us with a strong structural framework and to enable us to move our limbs in specific ways. The joints involve two forces acting in different directions, though some, such as our knees and elbows, are designed to bend in one direction only. In order for our joints to function well, they require strength and the ability to move and act effectively. Thus, if we take the metaphorical view, our personal strength, along with the ability to move our joints and perform as needed, can directly relate to our sense of worth.

If we are able to complete the tasks, run that race, climb that mountain, for example, then we will value ourselves highly in a society where productivity and success are often 'related' to what we're able to do.

Conversely, if we feel **unable to do** something or are not physically strong enough or flexible enough, e.g. we weren't able to reach something or move quickly enough to catch something – either literally or metaphorically - then it can leave us feeling as if our worth has been diminished. There are many studies to back this up, one of which I have

---

3   The cerebral cortex is "the outermost layer of your brain that contains six layers of nerve cells and is involved in many high-level functions, such as memory, thinking, learning, reasoning, emotion and senses." (https://my.clevelandclinic.org/health/articles/23073-cerebral-cortex)

referenced in the footnotes[4] however, the language in this article is a little technical so it may not be the easiest read.

In essence, different joints relate to different aspects of our lives. This means we can uncover clues about what is going on for us on an internal level if we look at which joint is affected. Going back to the situation with my knees, we know that knees are hugely important for us to walk and mobilise, and this is how we move forward. 'Moving forward' can metaphorically relate to moving forward in life or 'stepping up' to challenges, so when I later reflected on the pain I was experiencing in my knees, I realised there was a correlation - because I was also facing life challenges which at that time, felt insurmountable.

The more I explored this, the more I realised I was, in fact, feeling like Sisyphus in the Greek legend. Sisyphus was punished by Hades, the god of death, who forced him to roll an immense boulder up a hill. The problem was that whenever Sisyphus got close to the top of the hill, the boulder always rolled back down. This totally characterised my life at that time. For every two steps I took forward, I was taking three back, and so I dug deeper. I discovered, after more research, that knees can be suggestive of a 'sense of competition' and, as I often felt I wasn't good enough, I realised that the pain I was experiencing was my 'knees' communicating with me. I know that sounds odd, but this pain was, in actuality, a reflection of my perceived need to push myself ever harder to meet the expectations of others rather than listening to and addressing my own needs.

How our current health system fits into the picture (in relation to Loving)

When we become ill and go to the doctor, their response can have a profound effect on how we view our body and our symptoms. We can experience something called 'diagnostic shock', which can be so profound that it leads to our body developing further dis-ease. Then, when we are processing the prognosis or outcome (and remembering that we are by nature negatively wired), it can be all to easy to focus on the worst-case scenario. When we continue to entertain this pessimistic

---

4 If you'd like to read a case study exploring a condition affecting the bones – including the knee joints – follow this link: https://learninggnm.com/SBS/documents/Alvin_Case_95_E.pdf

view – as we've discussed at length throughout this book – it follows that this alone can affect how we are feeling and even contribute to the course of our dis-ease. In addition, we each have our own unique perspective and response to our illnesses, which might explain why conditions such as Parkinson's Disease and Multiple Sclerosis lead to severe deterioration in some people but not all. Taking this a stage further, can we argue that how we feel about ourselves determines our journey on the **thought-belief cycle**? We'll look at this in more depth later, but for now, it is important to recognise the power of our beliefs and inner voice and their associated impact.

AUTHOR NOTE: *The suggestion here is that we can see a causal link between our thoughts and beliefs and the physical impact on our bodies; however, I am not in any way advocating that appropriate medical advice should be ignored or not sought. My research and personal experiences have led me to conclude that our thought-belief system does have a noticeable impact on how we see both our wellbeing and our dis-ease, so my message is simply to be aware of this and consider how your own thoughts/beliefs may be contributing to your overall wellbeing. Then, if you find a link, it is important to address these when looking for ways to support healing in order to achieve the most desirable outcome. This complements any medical support rather than replacing it.*

Our inner voice is a reflection of the (sometimes toxic) culture in which we live. Fact?

Hopefully, you can now see how easy it is for us to entertain a critical inner voice and that this often escapes our notice because it has been with us forever and has become deeply embedded in our perceptions of ourselves. We can even think it's normal and natural to speak to ourselves this way.

Dr Maté, in his latest book, *'The Myth of Normal: Trauma, Illness and Healing in a Toxic Culture'*, looks at how our society's norms can be detrimental to our wellbeing, in particular where behaviours which are far from natural have become normalised. He contrasts our current busy, modern society with hunter-gatherer groups from centuries ago and shows how we have moved significantly away from how we were designed to live.

Whilst society has evolved, our basic human needs have remained static – genetically, we are just the same as we have always been. Yes, we have become highly 'domesticated' and 'conditioned' to the life we're living, but that doesn't mean it's good for our health and wellbeing. This idea has been explored extensively and is now reflected in various health statistics, such as the increase in dementia worldwide[5], the decreased 'healthy life expectancy' for women[6] and the continued increase in cancer diagnoses in the UK[7].

Also:

"The number of prescribed medicines supplied in primary care in England has increased steadily year on year. The total number of items dispensed in 2016 was over 1,104 million, an increase of 1.9% (20.5 million additional items) on the number dispensed in 2015. The average number of prescription items per head of the population in 2016 was 20.0, compared with 19.8 items in the previous year. The therapeutic area showing the greatest numeric rise since 2015 was antidepressants, with an increase of 3.7 million items (6.0%)".[8]

"The number of prescription items dispensed increased from 2006 to 2016 by 47%; the average number of prescription items per person per year has risen by 35% over this period from 14.8. The use of medicines to treat cardiovascular

5   https://assets.publishing.service.gov.uk/media/60c892108fa8f57ce980b6b7/GO-Science_Trend_Deck_-_Health_Section_-_Spring_2021.pdf
6   As reported in the Gov.uk Health Trend Deck for 2021
7   As discussed in this article from the UK Government: https://www.ons.gov.uk/peoplepopulationandcommunity/healthandsocialcare/conditionsanddiseases/bulletins/cancerregistrationstatisticsengland/2017#cancer-diagnoses-continue-to-increase
8   NHS Digital. Prescription Cost Analysis: prescriptions dispensed in the community, 2016. Leeds, NHS digital, 2017. www.gov.uk/government/statistics/prescription-cost-analysis-england-2016 . Note that cost at list price is the basic cost of a drug excluding VAT and is not necessarily the price the NHS paid. It does not take account of any contract prices or discounts, dispensing costs, fees or prescription charges income, so the amount the NHS paid will be different.

disease and respiratory disease has increased by 36% and 38% respectively over these 10 years, based on prescriptions dispensed in the community in England."[9]

"The year with the highest items dispensed [in England] was 2022/23, when 1.08 billion items were dispensed, a significant increase from the 850 million items dispensed 12 years previously."[10]

Bearing this in mind, I believe it's time to take a good, deep look at how we're living and make some radical changes if we want to feel happier and healthier and enjoy a more fulfilling life.

One could argue that the increase in diagnosis of illness and the prescribing of medication is due to the improvement of testing and screening and the increasing size and age of the population. There's also a concern that medical professionals are overprescribing[11] and using pills to treat symptoms rather than encouraging people to explore lifestyle changes. Even taking these factors into consideration, I still believe it would benefit our overall health if we were to get curious about this upward trend in the use of medication and ask ourselves:

- Why are we becoming a nation so reliant on pills and chemicals?
- Might there be a better way?
- How might we work with our bodies to maintain optimum health in natural ways for as long as possible?

Of course, as individuals, we might not be able to make changes on a large scale, but by exploring these questions in our own lives, we can develop a deeper understanding, make the changes that are right for us, and break the pattern of unconscious choices that might have been in place for generations, thus creating a better future for ourselves.

---

9   Taken from Health Survey for England 2016 Prescribed medicines http://healthsurvey.hscic.gov. uk/media/63790/HSE2016-pres-med.pdf

10   https://www.statista.com/statistics/418091/prescription-items-dispensed-in-england/

11   See 'Overprescribing of medicines must stop, says government', https://www.bbc.co.uk/news/ health-58639253

It's not inconceivable for this work we do on ourselves to have a ripple effect and touch the lives of our families, friends and work colleagues. If we put self-care at the top of our own agenda, if we love ourselves, it models this behaviour for others and helps them to see what a difference it can make. Not only that, but it permits them to do the same for themselves.

Self-care, therefore, isn't selfish; quite the opposite, it's the best gift we can give, both to ourselves and to those around us.

W·I·L·D® and Learning to Love Ourselves in a Practical Way

So, the big question is, how can we be more **loving** towards ourselves?

As I mentioned at the beginning of the chapter, we can start by getting curious and observing our inner voice, making sure we do this as gently as we can. We need to be deeply kind and compassionate with ourselves. It's not about beating ourselves up. It's about noticing how we speak to ourselves and understanding the extent of any criticism from our inner voice and how that makes us feel. This will help us to appreciate how detrimental this narrative is to our wellbeing and how much better we can feel when we reframe our inner dialogue to be more **loving** and supportive.

It can be useful to bear in mind that the reason we feel such discomfort when we listen to our inner critic is because what it's saying is out of alignment with what our Inner Nature knows to be true.

Personally, I interpret the degree of discomfort I feel when I listen to my inner critic as a metric for how much our Inner Nature believes it to be untrue. It is my belief that words like 'lazy' and 'stubborn' are labels we can take on board and cognitively believe; however, they probably aren't true 100%. We might have elements of these traits, but to label ourselves as entirely 'lazy' or 'stubborn' (or any other negative adjective) is unfair. Our inner voice doesn't make this distinction, though, and so it's down to us to notice and call this out. We do this by using our level of discomfort as our own internal 'lie detector'.

Would we label animals as lazy due to the amount of sleep they engage in? Perhaps we do sometimes, but I think this simply highlights our conditioned perception rather than stating fact. Sleep serves a purpose for all animals (including us), and every animal's needs vary depending upon their physiology and other factors. I personally think that (unhelpful) labels are often:

- other people's projections about things they don't like/find uncomfortable.

- reflections of where we don't feel safe.

- habits that serve some sort of purpose for us - though not necessarily beneficial ones.

When our 'lie-detector' is activated, and if we use this carefully, we can spot the false statements from our critical voice and start reframing them into something which helps us to feel a bit better. To start **Loving** ourselves more. At this point, I would recommend taking another look at the diagram below, which outlines different emotions and their vibration level.

Upward Spiral

THE EMOTION SCALE

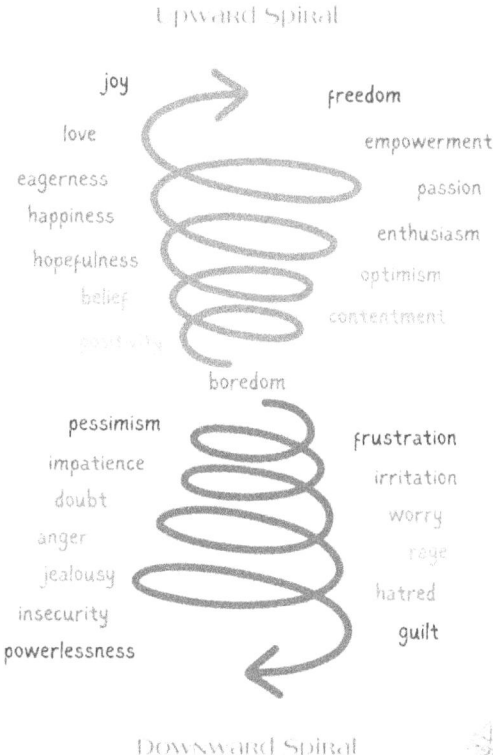

joy

love

freedom

eagerness

empowerment

happiness

passion

hopefulness

enthusiasm

belief

optimism

contentment

boredom

pessimism

frustration

impatience

irritation

doubt

worry

anger

rage

jealousy

hatred

insecurity

guilt

powerlessness

Downward Spiral

The higher its vibration, the more uplifting, liberating and healing that emotion will be. Lower vibrations are usually generated by emotions which are disempowering and can feel deeply uncomfortable or even painful.

Powerlessness is at the very bottom of the scale because it has the lowest emotional vibration. Feeling or being powerless can be incredibly difficult to manage and usually leads to a low mood and feelings of insufficiency.

As you travel up the vibrational scale, you pass through **guilt, insecurity, hatred, jealousy, rage, anger,** etc, which are also emotions often labelled as 'negative'. But if you think about it, these emotions are higher up the scale than powerlessness, so even if you are feeling jealous, for example, it is arguably a more hopeful emotion than powerlessness. That's not to say that these higher vibrational emotions are comfortable; it's just that any step upward is heading in the right direction.

You may well find these lower-vibration emotions uncomfortable, but if you refer back to this scale you can use it to help reframe that inner voice towards an emotion which moves you closer to where you want to be.

> **TIP:** Try 'reverse engineering' from the emotion you would like to achieve, to the emotion you are currently experiencing in order to figure out what you can do to move yourself closer to where you want to be. You can do this by reframing your thoughts to be more in alignment with the next level, and then the next, and the next, and so on.

In some situations, you might find yourself just above 'boredom' on the scale, for example, and taking steps to move up the scale from there will be relatively easy. For emotions that are below 'boredom', though, this might prove more of a challenge. The key here is to recognise where we are and, if we can, work out why. This can help us to realise that the struggles we have faced to move upwards exist for a (good) reason. And then, we can address these.

Depending on where your 'baseline' is on the scale, it might be realistic to expect to move up only one turn of the spiral, which might not feel a whole lot better at first. If, for example, we've gone from hatred to anger, we might not consider this to be an improvement. In fact, we might even find it difficult to distinguish between some of the emotions, which is where the Body Scan (see Chapter 5) and Emotion Wheel (in Appendix 6) can really help out. The Emotion Wheel in particular, helps us to develop a greater emotional literacy, enabling us to see and understand nuances between our emotions and thus consciously respond in healthy and appropriate ways. Having these tools available whilst doing any work on your emotions will provide a much better outcome than simply reacting out of unconscious conditioned patterns of behaviour.

To put this into a relatable context - suppose someone was feeling pessimistic about their relationship. If they spend time thinking about all the problems they're having with their partner, this could lead to frustration, irritation and impatience. These emotions may then cause them to doubt the value of the relationship. However, if they recognised that they were feeling pessimistic and looked at the Emotion Scale, they would see that pessimism is close to boredom. The pessimism they are feeling, thus, may simply indicate a need to inject more fun and spontaneity into their relationship. Focusing on this instead, they will feel a greater sense of positivity, hopefulness and optimism, along with an increased value in both their partner and relationship as a whole.

Changing our thought processes in this way puts the focus of control back on us. We are no longer looking for reasons for the concern in our relationship; instead, we are actively seeking to change our focus and thus achieve a positive outcome.

Alternatively, we may ultimately decide to end the relationship but at least we will be able to go through the process in a loving way, being true to ourselves and handling the separation as gracefully as possible. This benefits not only us but also everyone else involved. It might still be a sad and painful process, but hopefully a less traumatic one.

The more we focus on the things that make us happy, the more happy things we notice - because we've set our filters to pick up on these elements of our experience. A bit like filtering an internet search. If we filter out the sad and focus on the happy, momentum on our upward spiral is gained, and this, in turn, can more easily connect us with gratitude, love and a sense of freedom and joy. From this (emotional) place, life feels much more fulfilling, and we personally become empowered, energised and more creative and resourceful.

> **TIP:** It takes a minimum of 21 days to create a new habit. It takes a lot longer to break an old habit than it does to create a new one. The trick is to focus on the habit we want to create rather than worrying about the old habit we want to drop.

When we're aware of our self-talk and how it makes us feel, and when we know what our feelings are and where we want them to be on the emotion scale, then we can start exploring what we might say to ourselves to help us make that shift.

But remember, it's crucial to be patient with ourselves. Here is a mantra that you might find helpful:

Where our attention goes
our energy flows
and the object of our focus grows

Therefore, we need to put our energy into cultivating the new habit rather than fighting the old one.

Also, remember this rule:

What we resist persists!

This is another reason *not* to think about the old behaviours that we no longer want in our lives.

<u>Making it fun</u>

A way to make this process easier is to make it fun. Rather than getting annoyed or irritated with yourself, as if it was some sort of 'test' you failed, see it as a game. Laugh when you find yourself slipping back into the unwanted old habit and say something ridiculous like 'Whoops!' or any other word you care to use. For example:

- if your aim is to stop smoking, but you find yourself with a cigarette between your lips before you've even realised you've opened the packet – smile and say, 'Whoops!'
- if you're trying to eat more healthily, and you find yourself reaching for a doughnut from the box in the office kitchen – smile and say, 'Whoops!'
- if you've promised yourself that you'll address your inner critic, then suddenly realise that you've been beating yourself up internally for the last 10 minutes - smile and say, 'Whoops!'

If you are at any of these points or similar, it's time to do an 'about turn' and laugh with yourself. I sometimes think of this as a change of direction and say, 'Oops, plot twist!' This helps me to stop the old habit and take the opportunity to explore why I might have slipped back into it:

? **What was the trigger?**
  » Stress? Boredom? Feeling tired/anxious/unhappy?

? **What was my need at that moment?**
  » Energy? To feel a sense of comfort?

Once I'm clear on why I have slipped back into the old habit, then I can look for other, more supportive ways to address the need. The main thing is not to give up. See this not as a mistake but as an opportunity to start again. Wipe your metaphorical slate clean. And the good news is, you're not starting from scratch this time. Not only that, but you will also be more aware of what caused you to slip and perhaps how to catch yourself earlier next time. In doing this, you build up your skills and learn how to listen to your body's clues more intently.

Then, you can start to treat yourself with more ease, compassion and grace and become more Loving towards yourself.

The more you become conscious and stay conscious, the easier this process becomes, and not just because I am telling you it does, but because there is a sound physiological reason. Over the years, our brains become wired a certain way through repetition - imagine paths like deep grooves, ruts even, where we have trodden the same thought over and over again, leading to the walls of the ruts being steep and slippery. Like a crevasse. These steep and slippery sides can make it challenging to get out of these ruts, yet it's very easy to fall back in. This alone helps to explain why it's easier to create a new habit than to break an old one. The more we practice the new habit, the deeper those new grooves become, strengthening these new paths and connections. Often, before we know it, we can find this new behaviour happening automatically. The old grooves (behaviours) will then gradually fade away as they are no longer being maintained – think of weeds and trees growing over an untended path.

> **TIP:** Take a moment to think about this: When we are blindly living from conditioning (that has come from learnt behaviours or previous life experiences and habits), it can leave us feeling inadequate and deeply miserable. Especially if we are aiming for the current 'societal' values, which may not be in line with our True Nature. When we can recognise this and start to live in a way that is true for us as an individual rather than merely following the rest of society, then we can become confident, happy, fulfilled and at ease. What's more, our health will improve and don't forget, our behaviour will almost certainly rub off on those around us, too.

Something else that I've found really helpful, particularly during the times when I felt disconnected from my Self, was to look for inspiring role models. Who could I see embodying the values and practices that I aspired to? I could then use their example as a benchmark to discover if I was following my own heart or following the conditioning of society.

This is an exercise I continue to use regularly.

My personal role models have varied depending on where I am, what behaviours I'm addressing or what skills I want to develop at the time. They might be a character in a book or a film, someone in my network, a family member or friend, or a public figure. When life feels challenging in some way, I 'spend time' with one or more of these people – watching a movie, reading a book, networking, having a chat, watching YouTube videos, or whatever. This activity inevitably inspires and uplifts me, much like giving my car a tune-up and oil change, and I will set off again feeling refreshed and recharged.

Two of my favourites, whom I return to repeatedly, are *Brené Brown*, for her teaching on vulnerability, and *Gabor Maté*, for his teaching on compassion. Both I find to be deeply grounded, open and honest about themselves as well as their journeys and the challenges they've faced. This is something that I deeply respect.

In this way, they both embody the concept behind the 'L' of W·I·L·D®. They are a living example of what it means to love ourselves as we are and as we are not – that is, loving ourselves 'warts and all'. Embracing the 'shadow' aspects of ourselves and coming to see that even they (the shadows) have value and can contribute something of worth to our lives.

Back in Chapter 1, I referred to my 'stubborn streak'. Often, society teaches us that stubbornness is an unwanted trait. It's generally seen as a 'negative' label, yet it can stand us in really good stead at times. If you take Steve Jobs as an example here, he refused to listen to those who advised there would never be a time when personal computers were commonplace. Instead, he stuck to his guns and continued pushing forward with his vision. Without this stubborn streak, arguably, technology would not be as advanced as it is today.

Perhaps, then, it's not about labelling things 'right' or 'wrong', 'good' or 'bad', 'successes' or 'failures', but seeing every event, every experience, every emotion as a part of us and exploring how we can engage with them so that they serve us well, rather than make our lives unhappy, or worse, lead to dis-ease.

Chapter Summary

- We learned how loving ourselves is about accepting ourselves just as we are.

- Everyone is an amazing and beautiful being with their own unique gifts to share.

- Love is the highest of vibrations and enables us to experience a profound sense of joy and connection, which brings a sense of inner peace and wellbeing.

~ Eight ~

W·I·L·D®
D is for Dance

Inside Chapter Eight

The 'D' of W·I·L·D® is about seeing Life as a Dance. It brings together the concepts of Wonder, Intuition and Love to form a beautiful, graceful, joyful, supportive approach which we can use to help us navigate whatever life might throw at us. It's about finding our own personal rhythm and harmony in each moment and letting that guide and direct our steps. This is a magical alchemy enabling us to transform our fears into Love, Joy, Freedom and Wellbeing.

~ ~ ~ ~ ~

I have come to see Life as being like a dance – challenging, sure, but it can also be beauty-full, grace-full, and fun!

But this wasn't always the way. I used to see it more like a tough, uphill challenge, an unfair competition, or a fear-inducing test where I was being judged. And I saw that test as being pre-weighted against me, meaning I'd most likely fail.

However, through my journey and through exploring and engaging with the concepts of Wonder, Intuition and Loving myself, I came to realise that actually, Life doesn't judge us; Life isn't a competition. Life just seeks to experience, to learn and to grow, and in doing these things, it pursues living to its fullest. In exactly the same way as a Dance.

So, what changed for me?

When I realised that I was miserable, that's when I realised I needed to change my life because it was making me ill. In my worst moments, I felt unloved and unlovable, unwanted and that no one would care very much whether I lived or died. In my mind, it seemed as though everything always went wrong, and I generally believed life to be unfair.

When I began to research how I could change things and improve my life, I suddenly realised how much my 'thought habits' were contributing to how I was feeling. And that's when I thought about dancing.

Dancing is vibrant, full of light and colour, and it is joyful. All of these things were missing from my life, and the concept of dance encompassed what I was lacking so beautifully. With this in mind, I actively sought ways to view Life as the gift it is, rather than merely surviving day to day and, instead of struggling through each day and dreading the next, I began to look at my life as a Dance, a challenge that could be beautiful, graceful and fun.

I realise now that I used to take everything – including myself – so seriously. The problem with that is it led to my mind being closed, and my views narrowed, resulting in me becoming judgemental about everything that happened and never feeling as if I was 'good enough'.

> **IMPORTANT:** 'Good enough' is not a helpful metric to use. It is indefinable. There is no way to denote what constitues being 'good enough' or achieving 'perfection'. If we are striving to be 'good enough' based on other's achievements, then we are not being true to ourselves. The only person we need to be 'good enough' for, is ourselves.

Looking back, I can see now that I was using the wrong yardstick. I was looking outside of myself for validation rather than listening to my own heart, my True Nature, and letting that guide me. I was trying to follow someone else's rhythm rather than dancing to my own. I'd lost my tempo and harmony and fallen out of step with myself. In the words of Matshona Dhliwayo:

"Dance to the beat of your own drum;
whether the world likes your rhythmic movements or not."

As soon as I realised that I needed to 'dance to my own drum', that's when I reconnected with my sense of Wonder and Intuition and began to fall back in Love with me.

And that was when the magic happened. The intense pressure I had felt all of my life slowly began to ease.

There's a quote from Abraham-Hicks which always makes me smile:

"You all make too much of all of this!"

This is so true!

It's taken me a long time, but now I am able to see life as simply our own unique opportunity to explore and discover Who We Really Are and to live in accordance with our True Nature.

I understand this sounds simple – perhaps too simple – and you might have concerns that you won't be able to make these changes. You might be wondering how easy it is for you to make the same kind of adjustments and if you will be able to stick with them. Does this shift work for everyone?

The short answer is yes. Absolutely. I have simplified the process so that it can be accessible to all, but make no mistake, the work this involves is not always easy. Often, you will be going against the flow, maybe being a bit of a rebel or swimming against the tide, but if you trust your Intuition, allow yourself to explore in Wonder, Love yourself and give yourself permission to Dance along the way, you'll see changes that you never believed possible.

How can I be so sure?

It's simple.

There is a force stronger than all of our concerns, worries, and fears, and it is a force that every single one of us can tap into. Like the strength that comes from the pull and push of the ocean tide, we are all blessed with our own True Nature, our Life Force, and if we allow this to support and carry us, we can achieve anything, especially if we are willing to challenge societal norms.

When we can 'allow' and 'let be' – as Jack Kornfield put it – things will come and go as they're designed to, with much less effort, struggle or suffering on our part. As he said:

"To let go does not mean to get rid of. To let go means to let be. When we let be with compassion, things come and go on their own."

> **TIP:** Take a moment to re-read this quote and then really consider the message.
>
> What possibilities might you encounter if you did simply 'let be'?

When I think about and reference society and societal norms, I am inclined to agree with Dr Gabor Maté, who talks about the 'toxic culture' in which we live. In his book, *'The Myth of Normal: Trauma, Illness and Healing in a Toxic Culture'*, he states:

"I will make the case that much of what passes for normal in our society is neither healthy nor natural, and that to meet modern society's criteria for normality is, in many ways, to conform to requirements that are profoundly abnormal in regard to our Nature-given needs – which is to say, unhealthy and harmful on the physiological, mental and even spiritual levels…

When we can look soberly at what we as a culture have normalized about health and illness, and realize that is not, in fact, the way things are meant or fated to be, there arises the possibility of returning to what Nature has always intended for us."

Some of the beliefs that have become accepted as normal but which are not, in fact, healthy are reflected in comments I hear from people around me. Comments like:

- *'Push on through'*

  Don't. The messages from our body or our instinct might be telling us that we need to rest, recharge or rethink.

- *'Grin and bear it'*

  Stop. This can cause us to put up with situations that we actually find intolerable, meaning that we can end up dissociating from our feelings and putting our own needs at the bottom of the list.

- *'Think positive'*

  Impossible to achieve all the time and incredibly difficult to reach when we are feeling challenged or low. Don't get me wrong; I believe that it's helpful for us to focus on the positives and to look for them in any situation, but not in such a way that we sacrifice our wellbeing to do so. For me, it's more about finding a healthy balance. Forcing ourselves to put on a happy face when we're actually feeling deeply hurt, angry, sad or upset is not healthy. What we are doing is simply suppressing our emotions, which actually leads to depression and anxiety.

Remember: When we don't feel good, our body is giving us valuable information. This is the time to get curious and start exploring how we're feeling in more detail.

How do I do this?

If we go back to Dancing for a moment, imagine you're learning to dance for the first time – or learning a new style of dance that you haven't tried before. Initially, you might feel you have two left feet. You might struggle to pick up the rhythm and learn the steps. The volume of information you need to retain can seem overwhelming – what you should be doing with your left foot, what you should be doing with your right, what are your hands and arms supposed to be doing, your body, your head, your face? In time, though, and with practice, it gets easier. The parts start to come together and flow as a cohesive whole.

You will then relax, enjoy yourself and realise you're having fun. We can use the same process when it comes to our wellbeing. We can take time to learn each step and perfect each movement until we achieve the beauty of dance within ourselves.

◆ Exercise: Shall We Dance

Now that you've reached this point in the book, you may well have begun to listen to your Intuition and given more consideration to Loving yourself, but you don't know what to do next. You'd love to view your world with more Wonder but don't know how to experience the Dance – and I totally understand. It's a process, often of trial and error, but here's what I do:

To begin, I acknowledge that I don't feel good but I don't know what exactly that means. So, I ask myself a series of questions, something along the lines of:

- What is it about how I'm feeling that isn't how I'd like to be feeling?
- Can I say when this feeling started?
- Was it prompted by a particular event?
- What feelings did that event bring up for me?
- Or, if I can't pinpoint a specific event, do I have a sense of what the feelings relate to?
- What is it about the event or the situation that makes me feel uncomfortable?
- Is this the first time I've felt this way?
- If not, when have I felt it before?
- Is this current situation reminding me of a painful experience in my past?

I will take a good few minutes to do this – perhaps longer – and I always record the answers to my questions in a journal or notebook. It would be beneficial for you to do the same.

Asking questions like these and recording the answers in a journal or notebook or even a memo app on your phone, can help to bring insight, clarity and deeper self-understanding. Rather than being at the mercy of apparently nameless feelings which appear to arise out of nowhere, this practice will help to develop your emotional awareness and ability to put this into words. In turn, once we have found the words, we can then better express our feelings – which means not only communicating them (which plays a role in finding our place and 'our people' and making those valuable and healing connections) but also 'getting those feelings out'. This we can do by, for example, talking to others, friends, professionals and families, taking a walk, shouting from the top of a mountain, meditating, joining a group of like-minded individuals … all manner of outlets are there for us to use. Now that we have identified the feelings and the areas in which we are challenged, it is so much easier to find the most appropriate outlet – and there may be more than one – and then we can 'dance to the beat of our own drum'.

Some years ago, I went to an Alexander Technique workshop where the facilitator talked about what she called 'The Fred Astaire principle'. Fred Astaire was a famous dancer who appeared in several movies in the 1930s. He was known for his skill, grace and elegance and would glide across the floor, making it look effortless - but this didn't 'just' happen. It took him hours of practice, commitment and dedication, an effort he never minded because dancing was his passion. When he danced, he was having fun and bringing joy to all who watched him.

If we view our Life as a dance, something of a passion, we can begin to explore our own particular style, rhythm, harmony and grace in everything that we do. Ask yourself:

1. Are you someone who likes to be active and busy most of the time, or do you prefer to move at a slower, more reflective pace?

2. Do you like to be surrounded by people or to spend periods of time by yourself?

3. What makes you smile; what environments and activities do you most enjoy?

Listen to how you answer these questions and think about what you can do and what adjustments you can make to bring what you need into your life. If you work in a busy office, for example, yet find noise overwhelming, perhaps it's worth exploring a different way of working.

In life, we can feel clumsy and uncoordinated. We have so much to be aware of, to juggle and manage at the same time, yet if we take it one step at a time and listen to our own inner guidance and tempo, we'll find our rhythm and, like the dancing, we will start to enjoy ourselves.

And the best part is, when we find our own beat, our joy will ripple out and light up the lives of those around us, inspiring them to join in in their own unique way.

Chapter Summary

- We discovered how to see life as a Dance.
- I illustrated how doing this will make it easier for you to experiment and try new things.
- We learned how important it is to 'let life happen'.
- We discussed the benefit of learning new skills but doing so without any fear or trepidation.
- We realised that if we put unreasonable expectations on ourselves (which may be based on societal norms), ultimately, this can be detrimental.
- Dance is all about having fun!

~ Nine ~

W·I·L·D® The Psychology
Is Ignorance really Bliss?

Inside Chapter Nine

In this chapter, we will dig deeper into the psychology of forming new habits, and I will provide you with tools to assist in reshaping your perspective and routines into something more uplifting and healing.

~ ~ ~ ~ ~

Up until this point in our lives, we may have been unaware of everything that is still out there for us to learn. In many ways, we may have been living in 'blissful ignorance' of our lack of knowing. In the 1970s, Noel Burch referred to this as *'Unconscious Incompetence'* in Gordon Training International's "four stages for learning any new skill" (*Wikipedia) - https://en.wikipedia.org/wiki/Four_stages_of_competence*.

The word 'incompetence', however, can have negative connotations so I've chosen to reframe this slightly and to talk about it as a state of 'unknown not-knowing' as illustrated by the diagram below.

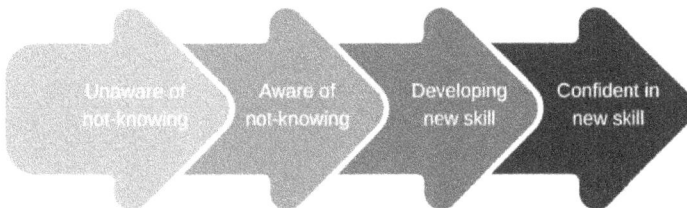

Unaware of not-knowing → Aware of not-knowing → Developing new skill → Confident in new skill

FOUR STAGES OF COMPETENCE

Setting out on this journey of W·I·L·D® exploration will bring us up against all sorts of new experiences and information that we are unaware of not knowing, which can be daunting. Suddenly, when we realise how much we don't know, we are left with a choice. We can either:

a. see this as an opportunity to explore further, embrace those new thoughts, feelings and experiences, try them out for size and see what they might have to teach us,

or

b. decide that it's not for us, back away and retreat to our 'safe' place where we were before.

Taking the first option, we might, for example, discover a talent we didn't know we had or a career we'd never considered, and this leads us to the next stage in the process – *we become aware of not knowing*. From here, we can make a conscious choice to learn and grow. If, though, we take option (b), we will stay exactly where we are and risk missing out on new and wonderful opportunities.

When we choose to engage in developing a new skill, it's important to understand that it will take time for us to become familiar with it and to start putting it into practice. It's not yet a habit so the steps we are taking may feel awkward and clunky.

REMEMBER: It takes at least 21 days to start building a new habit AND there's a better chance of success if you focus on creating the new habit rather than dropping the old one. Our mind will happily provide us with all manner of reasons to avoid the new behaviour though, so beware. Excuses like, it's late, you're tired, you've had a hard day at work, you don't have the right clothes, you've never done this before so you won't be any good at it ... and so on. At this point, you need to make a choice not to listen to your mind and instead promise yourself that you will make self-care a priority, no matter how you feel, because you value yourself and your wellbeing.

So, we're developing a new skill, but we're not yet as proficient as we'd like to be, which can be an uncomfortable place emotionally. We are in that seesaw of, *'I'm doing well considering I've only just started learning'* yet, at the same time, *'Why is everyone else dancing so much better than me?'*

What is crucial here is to note that we're moving from **awareness of our not-knowing towards development of the new skill**. We are going along that line **towards being confident** in our new skill, but we are doing it in our own time – which is perfectly okay. In fact, this is to be encouraged. If we do it in our time and at our pace rather than measuring our achievements against others, we will be progressing with compassion and consideration towards ourselves rather than being weighed down by the burden of unrealistic expectations.

In time, the new practice will become second nature, and we will no longer need to think about it as much. We will have become confident in our new skill. When we reach this point, we have arrived at 'competence' because this skill is now subconscious – it has become embedded in our muscle memory - and we will (a) be more confident in using it and (b) use it without realising it.

Think about when you first started learning to drive, for example. Initially, it might have felt like an impossible task with too many things to remember and do at the same time. You need to be watching the road whilst also obeying any signs, traffic lights or crossings. You have to be aware of cyclists and pedestrians whilst at the same time looking in your mirrors, using the indicators, working the pedals, changing gear and steering. It sounds overwhelming, and at the beginning, it is. All of these actions feel separate and disjointed. The more you practice driving, though, the more the skill evolves, and you start to build muscle memory. Soon, you stop having to think about each step individually because it becomes more natural, and in no time at all, they flow as one. It's no longer a case of 'mirror – signal – manoeuvre'. Instead, it becomes one smooth action of driving.

Habits are exactly the same. When I first decided to go for a walk in our local park every day, I struggled - particularly in the winter months.

I'd make excuses: it was too cold/wet/dark; I was too tired; work had been stressful, and I just wanted to sit and rest. But I knew that it was important for my wellbeing, so I made walking every day a 'non-negotiable' – something that I would not accept excuses for but would carry on and do it no matter how much I might not feel like it. This worked well, and in time, I came to appreciate my walks no matter what the weather was like because I could feel the difference they were making to my wellbeing. When I started to feel the difference, that's when I knew that I'd successfully created a new habit which was bringing me so many benefits. There was no way I was going back to how things were before.

The same is true for every new skill, so when we start to build a new self-care practice, it takes time for us to develop a sense of flow here, too. Whether our self-care practice is a commitment to go for a walk in Nature every day, to meditate, or to make time for mindfulness or journaling, it can feel alien at first. It might also feel outside of our comfort zone. When this happens, one thing you can do is explore how to bring in a sense of play and fun and take away some of the pressure. The new habit or skill is not about doing what you 'should'; it's simply an experiment to see if it supports your sense of wellbeing. The more fun it is, the more likely you are to engage with the new activity and thus build the habit.

Journal your discoveries

As I've mentioned before, journaling your thoughts and feelings is hugely beneficial and will help you to see them from a new perspective. Putting them down on paper and allowing them to flow through your pen – or keyboard if you prefer – helps you to see things from a different, more objective angle, as well as helping you to see the bigger picture. When you have things written down, it is also easier to clarify and explore the pros and cons of any given situation as well as discovering any patterns in your life which are constantly repeating. Journaling gives you the space, time and permission to ask the deeper questions that you might not have looked at thus far.

Remember: Emotions can be uncomfortable, BUT that's okay. They have important information to share with us when we give them space and expression so as long as we remember to stay curious and compassionate, then we can allow these to flow gently without pushing, forcing or resisting them.

W·I·L·D® in practice

It's worth remembering that Life is a dynamic, constantly moving force, and if we aren't consciously adjusting in response, we can experience a sense of being left behind. Similarly, it may be stronger and faster than we are prepared for, and it could be taking us in a direction of which we're unsure, somewhere that we don't feel comfortable.

A new career, for example, could be both a positive step and anxiety-inducing. We might, therefore, decide that it's easier to continue as we are rather than deal with the emotions associated with the change. Whilst this is perfectly understandable, I generally believe that we owe it to ourselves to make our choices consciously and for ourselves. This includes those which are outside of our comfort zone. If we really tune into our True Nature, as we have been discussing throughout this book, then our gut will tell us which steps we need to take and if these feel difficult, that's okay. We just need to remember to take it gently.

If we avoid making choices or leave them in the hands of others, we are giving away our response-ability, which can ultimately lead to us losing our sense of power and control over our own life. And that's the key. It's OUR life.

☆ Tips for putting W·I·L·D® into practice:

★ Where possible, take a moment of pause before making a choice. Use this time to observe and listen to your Intuition before deciding on the next steps.

★ Make any decisions consciously, i.e. reflect on your own needs, wants and desires.

★ Show patience and compassion towards yourself – regardless of the decisions you make and their resulting actions.

★ Give yourself permission to put your own needs first. This is the only way that we can truly discover who our 'best self' is.

★ Remember that what you are doing here will be wonderfully supportive for your own wellbeing, and that will ultimately spread to those around you.

★ Put aside old, long-held beliefs that are no longer serving you. This can be challenging, so I have dedicated the next section to this point alone.

Putting aside old beliefs

Putting aside old, long-held beliefs – even when we know they're no longer serving us – can be challenging. As an example, one of my previous beliefs was to stick with things that felt safe and familiar to me in an effort to keep myself protected and avoid potential harm. Whilst there's nothing wrong with this belief, it became a habit, a default. I found my world getting smaller and smaller over time because as soon as I bumped into the edge of my comfort zone, I backed away. That led to fear, which made me move to reduce the size of my comfort zone even further. It was a vicious circle.

When I started to reflect more deeply on this I realised that rather than helping me to feel safer, this behaviour actually made me more fearful of the situations I was avoiding because I was building them into something increasingly scary. Realising this, I started to stretch myself - very gently at first. I would do simple things like taking my regular walk in the opposite direction, trying out a different recipe, or creating new outfits from my wardrobe, just to see how it felt and to show myself that it's okay to try fresh things. As a result, I discovered that not only did the world continue to turn, but sometimes I found that I preferred this 'new' way of doing things.

It didn't always happen that way, though. There were times when the experience just felt 'different', and occasionally, I found the new option didn't work so well – but that was okay. I had given it a go, stretched my comfort zone, and realised that it had been safe for me to do so all along. The belief I had was, therefore, totally redundant.

Identifying unhelpful beliefs and behaviours

To identify beliefs and behaviours which are no longer serving us we need to look for those that lead us into repeating unhelpful patterns. In my teens, for example, I developed an unhelpful behaviour where, when I felt stressed, I would push myself too hard. I went into 'fight or flight', lost my appetite, and only picked at my food. Clearly, this pattern is incredibly detrimental over time, and it led (for me) to exhaustion, frayed nerves and unhealthy weight loss.

Common examples of unhelpful habits include:

- Procrastination – because you'll never get anywhere.

- Being constantly busy and never taking time to rest – because you'll be exhausted.

- Putting ourselves down all the time and being unable to accept compliments –reinforces any negative beliefs we hold about ourselves.

- Ignoring issues that we know need our attention, allowing them to escalate – because they become even more challenging to deal with in the long run.

Some unhelpful behaviours – such as dependency on alcohol, drugs, sex, gambling or shopping - can also be recognised as addictions, and it's worth realising here that the actual definition of addiction has a wider application than we perhaps first think:

"Addiction involves:
1. compulsive engagement with the behaviour, a preoccupation with it;
2. impaired control over the behaviour;
3. persistence or relapse, despite evidence of harm; and

4. dissatisfaction, irritability or intense craving when the object – be it drug, activity or other goal – is not immediately available."[1]

From this, we can see that it's not so much the behaviour itself that causes the problem, but more our relationship to it.

One of the most common unhelpful beliefs that I have encountered is *'I'm not worthy'* or *'I'm not good enough'*, and these are just two of the beliefs that drive imposter syndrome and lack of confidence. If you tune in to how this belief/statement feels in your body, you'll notice that its energy is low down on The Emotion Scale. I recommend referring to this Scale regularly and testing your feelings against it, as this will enable you to easily detect beliefs that aren't serving you. If you're feeling an emotion on the lower part of this scale, for example, you'll generally discover there's an unhelpful belief behind it.

Once you've discovered the belief, you can take action to reframe it. This will help you move higher up the scale and start to feel closer to those uplifting, joyful emotions that will make you feel more at home in your own skin.

How do we reframe beliefs?

One simple, but highly effective way in which we can start to reframe our beliefs is to use a 'Focus Wheel'[2].

Exercise: The Focus Wheel

1. Start by getting a blank piece of paper and drawing the diagram on the opposite page.
2. Now, choose an aspect of your life that you'd like to change – a thought, belief or sensation which currently leaves you feeling uncomfortable or unhappy – for example, "I'm rubbish at speaking in public", "I hate the way I look" or "My back is so painful". This becomes the

---

1   In the Realm of Hungry Ghosts, Gabor Maté, Chapter 11, 'What is Addiction'
2   An exercise shared by Abraham-Hicks – see https://www.youtube.com/watch?v=Vv_DBfgLhjM

title for your Focus Wheel. Don't spend too long on this part of the exercise, though. It's important to go where your intuition takes you and not overthink it. Otherwise, you could talk yourself out of it or end up down a rabbit hole, neither of which would be beneficial.

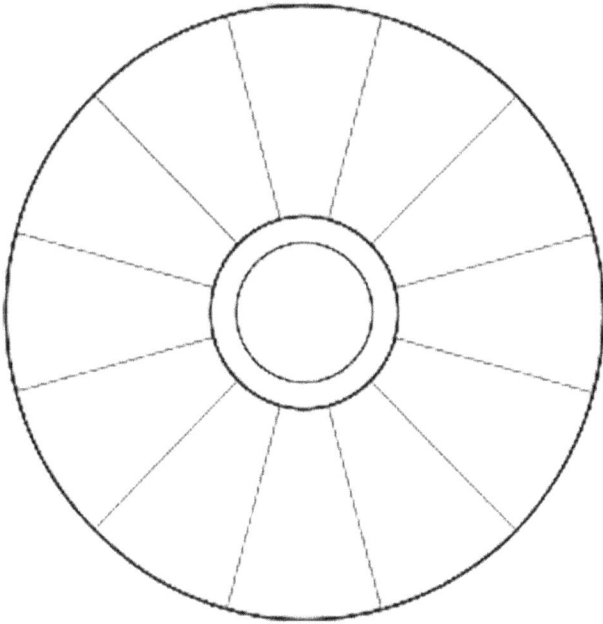

3. Once you have your title, think about how you would like things to be different. What your end goal is, perhaps? If you are concerned about public speaking, for example, you could reverse your negative comment to, "I'm an inspirational speaker, and audiences engage deeply with what I have to share". With body confidence, you could say, "I love my body and rejoice in how it looks and feels", or "I enjoy complete freedom of movement and feel totally at ease and comfortable in my body". Once you're happy with this new statement, write it in the central circle of your diagram.

4. You will now have a title written above your circle and a positive statement written in the centre.

5. The next step is to find thoughts and beliefs which relate to your central statement that you don't disagree with.

This is important. You want these thoughts and beliefs to be something you can say to yourself without feeling an inner niggle of doubt or disagreement.

6. To help with this, imagine your wheel is like a merry-go-round, and it's spinning at a constant speed. In order to get onto the wheel, the thoughts or beliefs you create need to be at the same speed; otherwise, they won't be able to get onto your wheel and, as Abraham-Hicks would say – will be "spun off into the bushes".

7. This first statement is going to be the hardest, and remember, you need to be able to say it to yourself without feeling a niggle of doubt or disagreement. Let's take the public speaking example to illustrate.

8. At first, it will be too much to make a statement as bold as "People flock to hear me speak" – that will be too uncomfortable, so instead, look for something that feels more relatable. Perhaps you can reflect on a time when you spoke to a friend about a book you had read and enjoyed, and they listened intently before asking to borrow the book. Whilst speaking to one person is very different to a group in a public speaking environment, this is still a great example of you inspiring someone with your words and engaging your audience in an effective way. Making a statement around this, "I can speak positively to others about books that I enjoy," for example, is increasing your speed closer to that at which your wheel is spinning, and thus, this statement can jump on board.

9. Now you have your first statement, write it in the top segment of your wheel. You will now have a title, a statement in the centre and one in the top segment.

10. It's time to think of another statement which feels true for you and builds on where you have started. Perhaps you could say, "I love meeting and speaking to new people." When you have this statement, it goes into the second segment, then build on this with a third. "I'm passionate

about my subject, and I love to share it with others," for example. This goes in the third segment, and so on.

11. Now you're on a roll. You're building your momentum, increasing your speed and raising your vibrational frequency – all of which takes you ever closer to the statement at the centre of your wheel. The goal is to achieve within yourself the vibrational frequency attached to that first statement. Building up in this way makes the transition from where you are to where you want to be much more manageable.

12. When all twelve segments of your wheel have been completed, tune in to how you're feeling now and notice the difference between this and how you felt at the start of the exercise. You'll probably find that your excitement level has risen, and you are much more ready to believe the statement at the centre of your wheel.

13. Finally, create a new statement to represent this feeling and write it in the circle around the central hub of the wheel. This is your re-framed belief.

14. You might like to write this re-framed belief on some sticky notes and put them where you'll see them easily and regularly. Each time you read them, feel the energy of this new belief and allow it to become a part of you. Also, if you catch yourself thinking the old thought, know that this is okay. The neural pathways for that thought will take time to fade away. Just congratulate yourself on noticing – this in itself is a huge step and a sign that you're doing really well - and gently shift your focus back to the new belief, thus building and strengthening this new neural pathway.

Sometimes, we can find ourselves experiencing more than one emotion at a time – perhaps even from different ends of the scale. It is possible, for example, to feel both happy and sad, enthusiastic and impatient, hopeful and doubtful, along with many other combinations. Though this may seem strange, it's perfectly normal. As humans, we have the capability to hold beliefs that are in opposition to each other and on different parts of the Emotion Scale. However, holding two opposing emotions can lead to unconscious, unhelpful behaviours such as procrastination.

For example, you might believe you are good at what you do, yet also have a deep-seated fear that you are not good enough. You then go around in circles worrying about all of the potential red flags, and before you know it, you're procrastinating. This then becomes a new habit, and you're rapidly heading in an unhelpful direction.

> **TIP:** If you find yourself juggling opposing emotions, simply pause and take a moment to consider what they are and then note them down. Think about what may have triggered them, what was happening in your day at the time and note this down too. Eventually you may notice patterns in your behaviour, which will help you to gain an awareness of what is going on. Then you can make adjustments, perhaps doing the Focus Wheel exercise, for example. You can also use these observations to help you identify and practice new behaviours which feel more supportive, uplifting and congruent with your True Nature.

True Nature – What is it?

Let's take a moment to re-visit our understanding of True Nature and what it is. Essentially, when we talk about True Nature, we are referring to 'who we really are' or 'the person we were born to be'. Often, this is not obvious, so for me, it's about taking on board all of the elements we have covered so far and working out how they apply. Many of the exercises will encourage you to dig deep and really listen to your body and inner self, which can seem daunting. But, when you really tune in, trust me, you will be rewarded with an incredible sense of calm because when we spend the time really breaking down our wants, desires and needs, that's when we will discover our True Nature.

Sometimes, though, life is just messy, and this can feel as if a tide of emotion is carrying us away with no map or compass. Navigating these strong waves is exhausting, even for the most resilient of us – just like being caught in a rip tide – and the danger here is that if we don't learn how to swim, we can experience emotional drowning, overwhelm and potential dis-ease. The key, if this is happening to you, is to go with the flow and not resist – exactly as you would in a rip tide.

How to navigate an emotional 'rip tide':

1 - Stay Calm:

√   Remember to breathe!

√   Avoid struggling or resisting the emotions.

√   Stay present; just observe what's happening within.

2 - Seek Support:

√   Don't hesitate to ask for help. Like summoning assistance in the water, sharing your feelings with someone can make a significant difference.

3 - Go WITH the Current:

√   Remember, e-motions are 'energy in motion.' They are ever-changing and evolving. Acknowledge that whatever you're feeling is temporary.

√   Instead of swimming against the emotional tide, consider floating until it passes or swimming across it, not against it, until you reach the calmer edge.

Understanding that emotions, like tides, are in constant motion helps us realise that whatever we're experiencing will pass in time, leaving things feeling calmer once more.

Chapter Summary

- We explored the challenges of putting aside old habits and replacing them with new, more supportive practices.
- We understood how to do this and the importance of building new and positive habits.
- We learned how to:
    » reframe unhelpful beliefs
    » navigate challenging emotional tides.

~ Ten ~

Bringing It All Together
Meta Consciousness®

Inside Chapter Ten

This section shares the learning which brought everything together for me. It was through Meta Consciousness® that I really developed a deeper understanding of, and healthier relationship with, my body, so it is important for me to share it with you here. This learning has also taken away my fear of dis-ease and given me the tools I need to work with my body, rather than fighting against it.

~ ~ ~ ~ ~

Now that we have completed our W·I·L·D® journey, I'd like to share one final element that really brought everything together and helped me understand what was happening in my body, why, and how to turn things around. This approach is called Meta Consciousness®.

Meta Consciousness® is like a multi-coloured umbrella which connects all the spokes of what I've learnt from working with animals, my love of Nature, my fascination with energy and emotion, as well as my reading of Eckhart Tolle, Gabor Maté, Bruce Lipton, Wayne Dyer, Louise Hay, Brené Brown and all the others (my umbrella has a lot of spokes!)

It sounds great, but what is Meta Consciousness®?

Simply put, Meta Consciousness® acknowledges that, as humans, we are just another form of mammal. We have the same basic emotions, needs and drives as all other mammals; the only real difference is that our cerebral cortex is generally larger (relative to our body size), which enables us to manipulate our environment to a greater extent than most other mammals. It also means that we can plan and create in a way other animals don't tend to, but having a larger cerebral cortex can have its downsides, too. For example, we are more prone to anxiety and depression and can also suffer from things like impostor syndrome and 'monkey mind' chatter. Yet, despite these differences, the similarities between us and all mammals on Earth are astonishing.

Dr Ryke Geerd Hamer, founder of German New Medicine (GNM, also known as German Healing Knowledge - GHK), was the man behind the roots from which Meta Consciousness® evolved. Dr Hamer carried out studies of cancer (following his own experience of prostate cancer), which led to him proposing a set of 5 Biological Laws. These laws, he believed, applied to all animals, including humans.

Through his work and research, Dr Hamer discovered something quite astonishing: 'Dis-ease' manifests and unfolds in all mammals by following the 5 Biological Laws he proposed:

Law One

Every dis-ease originates from an experience that we perceive as:

Unexpected[1]
Dramatic
Isolating[2], *and for which we have*
No coping strategy.

In Meta Consciousness®, we refer to this as a UDIN. The impact (energy) of these UDINs hits us first in the heart, then our brain and finally our body, with the whole process taking a matter of microseconds. The precise location in our body is determined by the nature of the shock.

---

1   *That is, it shocks us to the core. This can happen even if we think we should have been able to predict something – such as the death of a loved one or diagnosis of a serious illness.*
2   *Meaning that we feel alone in the situation and that we don't feel able to talk to anyone about it.*

What is important to note is that a UDIN is a *subjective* perception of an event. Two people in the same event might have very different experiences, which can result in different outcomes for their bodies, even though the situation is the same.

Our responses to these UDIN experiences can be both literal and metaphorical. In the microsecond of reaction time that it takes the body to analyse the energy of the UDIN, it will determine which organ, or organ tissue, is most appropriate for dealing with the issue, dependent upon the function of that organ or tissue.

For example, an animal may swallow a fragment of bone. If that fragment is too big to pass through the stomach, the stomach will respond by making extra acid-producing cells in order to facilitate the breakdown of the bone. The animal's body has recognised an 'undigestible morsel' and acted accordingly.

Humans, with our larger cerebral cortex and greater ability for metaphorical thinking, can experience this same physical response to other forms of 'indigestible morsels'. If you think about it, we link information to food in our everyday language, so the parallels can be drawn between an indigestible food morsel and indigestible information. Here are some examples:

- 'I bit off more than I could chew.'
- 'It left a bad taste in my mouth.'
- 'I couldn't swallow the news.'
- 'I couldn't stomach what they said.'
- 'I just couldn't digest the information.

When we use phrases like this, we are subconsciously helping our body to identify the organs and tissues which are trying to support us in processing the UDIN we have experienced. Therefore, if we listen to our language at the time of an event, it can be a massive clue as to where our body will send the energy we need to deal with the UDIN.

Some other phrases you might come across:

- 'I didn't want to see what was going on.' - eyes
- 'Something smelt off.' - nose/sinuses
- 'Shouldering a heavy burden.' – shoulders and back
- 'I wasn't strong enough.' – emotional and physical strength
- 'I was expected to bend over backwards.' – back and emotional flexibility

You can probably think of many more.

How do these parts of our bodies then respond?

This will depend on the affected tissue and its function. The diseases and symptoms we experience are not random. It's important to remember that our body isn't going wrong, making a mistake or attacking itself, it's simply trying to deal with a challenge in the best way it knows how. It's making adaptations to process the energy of the UDIN in order to survive and in order to learn, grow stronger and be better able to deal with any similar challenges it might face in the future.

What's happening in the brain?

The UDIN will also impact our brains, and here, the location of impact is determined by embryology.

When an egg is fertilised and begins to divide, it initially forms three different types of 'germ' cells: the *ectoderm*, *mesoderm* and *endoderm*.

All tissues of the fully formed body are derived from one of these three cell types, which means that these cell types can be used to classify our brain tissues (or layers) as well as the tissues and organs of the body that these brain tissues relate to.

The Brain Stem, for example, is the most primitive part of our brain and is made up of endodermal cells. These cells also make up much of our digestive tract, hence why the brain stem and our digestive systems are so closely linked.

Remarkably, it is actually possible to see where a UDIN has impacted our brain by studying a CT scan. UDINs show up on CT scans as a set of concentric circles that look like a target.

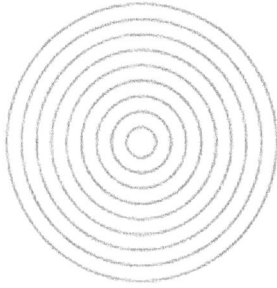

Law Two

Every dis-ease will go through two distinct phases to ensure that it reaches a full resolution.

Until then, if the UDIN shock is reactivated, the process of going through these phases remains ongoing.

These two phases are known as the Stress Phase and the Regeneration Phase. We can identify which phase we're in currently by how we feel:

- During the Stress Phase, we often don't feel ill. We are in a state of 'fight or flight' and operating in survival mode. Here, we can't afford to get sick! How could we fight for our lives or run for safety if we were feeling ill, exhausted and achy? Instead, our body pumps hormones such as adrenaline and cortisol to help numb our pain and give us the energy we need to beat or escape the threat. During this phase, we might feel restless, our feet and hands may be cold and clammy, and our mind may be overactive, which in turn leads to difficulty sleeping.

- When we are able to release the stress – either completely or to a sufficient degree – then our body goes into the Regeneration Phase. This is where we experience most of what we consider to be symptoms of dis-ease, such as aches and pains, inflammation, nausea, rashes, fatigue, fevers and so on. We get those 'flu-like symptoms' and want to take to our beds. These are signs that the body's natural healing processes are coming into play, and this is the point at which it's important for us to listen to our body. When we give ourselves permission to rest, to look after ourselves and allow the dis-ease to run its course, our bodies can, given the right conditions and vitality, return to full health once more.

Law Three

Dis-ease themes can be identified.

A theme is created based on where the original shock was registered both in the brain and in the body, which determines the adaptations our body undergoes along with the symptoms we experience.

As I mentioned earlier, when we experience a UDIN shock, it will hit our heart initially before being sent to the brain and then the body almost simultaneously. The UDIN energy is now, therefore, connected to both a tissue in the body and that tissue's corresponding area of the brain.

Tissues relating to different brain layers respond in different ways. In some tissues, this means creating extra cells to expand and increase the effectiveness of that tissue – like when the animal produces extra acid to aid digestion of the bone fragment. In other tissues, the body will go through a process of cell loss as a means of reducing the function of that tissue - for example, with the skin, in order to feel less. This can happen in the case of a touch that is wanted but not currently present (perhaps a child missing hugs from their mum) or an unwanted touch that the person currently feels unable to get rid of (such as in a physically abusive relationship). This is dependent upon the function of the tissue and the way in which the body is seeking to process the experience.

Our body is a very bio-logical system. By its nature, it is always seeking to adapt, learn and grow. When it experiences a UDIN, it recognises that this, too, is a learning opportunity. Sometimes, our body cannot access a suitable coping strategy at the exact moment of the event, so it will hold the shock within its tissues until it can find and employ a suitable strategy. We are also very metaphorical beings, and so our stomach might hold the issue if it's something we've found hard to digest or if it's something we want to run away from but feel unable to do so, our leg muscles will take this on and make adaptations until we can resolve the issue. This can, in part, explain why we feel tension in our necks from an unrelated stressor. Once a strategy has been developed and learnt, our body can then add it to its toolkit for future reference.

Law Four

Microbes[3] (things like bacteria) play an active and supportive role in the healing process.

And, by extension, our wellbeing.

It took me a long time to get my head around this; after all, we generally understand microbes to cause sickness and disease, so how can they possibly be something that supports the healing process?

In order to understand this, we need to take a look at our current medical system, which is based on a principle known as **Germ Theory**. This theory was proposed by Louis Pasteur, a French chemist and microbiologist, in the late 1850s who stated that '*diseases are caused by microorganisms known as pathogens or "germs"'*.

At around the same time that Pasteur proposed his theory, a fellow member of the French Academy of Science, Antoine Béchamp, put forward an alternative theory known as the **Terrain Theory.** Terrain theory states that *"if the body is well and balanced, then germs that are a natural part of life and the environment will be dealt with by the body without causing sickness".[4]*

---

3   *"Microbes are tiny living things that are found all around us and are too small to be seen by the naked eye." (https://www.ncbi.nlm.nih.gov/books/NBK279387/) Oxford Languages defines a microbe as "a microorganism, especially a bacterium causing disease or fermentation." (https://languages.oup.com/)*
4   *https://www.nutritionist-resource.org.uk/memberarticles/germ-theory-vs-terrain-theory-in-relation-to-the-coronavirus*

He argues further that we evolved alongside these microbes, so if they really were deadly killers, wouldn't they have wiped us out millennia ago? Or, to put it another way, how did we survive in the first place, before the presence of doctors, hospitals or pharmaceutical drugs, if, as Pasteur argues, germs are the real killers and we had no means to fight them?

> **Author Note:** *It is not my intention here to say one theory is right and the other wrong, merely to highlight the impact of perspectives on our beliefs and, therefore, on our practices and approaches. There are many factors at play in our overall wellbeing and our life expectancy. For me, the W·I·L·D® approach is about exploring and discerning to see what resonates with us as an individual and to use our power of choice to best support our wellbeing. The purpose of this book is simply to acknowledge the existence of both. There are many reasons why we enjoy a longer life expectancy now, including and irrespective of the improvement in drugs and medication. I have shared these as **theories** and included them to be read and interpreted as beneficial knowledge, which, I believe, adds to the whole W·I·L·D® journey. Anything beyond what I have written is outside of my understanding and, therefore, not within the scope of this book.*

Terrain Theory suggests that if our body (that is, our Mind-Body-Spirit-self) and the environment in which we live are robust and healthy, we will experience a high level of vitality. Because our 'terrain' is strong.

Consider for a moment how we live now, which is often in a state of high emotional stress. Correlate this to the number of people who experience chronic ill health and those who take prescription medicines on a daily basis. If Béchamp's argument is sound, could it be said that by changing our terrain, we can reduce those instances of chronic ill health or, indeed, the volume of prescribed medications?

I stated at the beginning that our medical system is based on Germ Theory, despite both Theories being postulated around the same time.

Reports suggest that although *"Béchamp was the more brilliant thinker, Pasteur had political connections, including Emperor Napoleon III. ... and he, Pasteur, achieved fame and fortune largely because his views 'were in tune with the science and the politics of his day.'"*[5]

Whatever the reason, Pasteur's theory was adopted by the medical profession and has become the accepted perspective ever since.

Interestingly, on his deathbed, Pasteur is alleged to have said:

"The microbe is nothing. The terrain is everything."

Based on these conflicting theories, it is valid, in my opinion, to consider that we may have things the wrong way around. Yes, we know that microbes are present in diseased tissue, but are they the cause of the dis-ease? If microbes are constantly around us in our environment – including on our skin and within our bodies – but we're not constantly sick, how then can we say they are to blame when we do fall ill? Might this be like blaming the fire brigade for the fire?

Meta Consciousness® teaches that the types of microbes found in tissues are specific to the origin of those tissues (i.e., whether they derived from the endoderm, mesoderm or ectoderm layer). Also, these microbes act in particular ways to help undo the Stress Phase adaptations and to restore balance and homeostasis to the body.

What this means in effect is:

- Where cells *increase* during the Stress Phase, microbes help to break these cells down, which can cause pus and bleeding to appear during the Regeneration Phase.
- Where cells *decrease* during the Stress Phase, microbes help to rebuild the cells by filling in holes and making the tissues strong once more. In this instance, the microbes become our 'restoration crew' and support our healing.

---

5 *https://www.westonaprice.org/health-topics/notes-from-yesteryear/germ-theory-versus-terrain-the-wrong-side-won-the-day/#gsc.tab=0*

This is why overuse of antibiotics is not a good thing because antibiotics are designed to kill off bacteria, which means that they effectively remove our clean-up and restoration crews.

You might be wondering how this relates to the recent experience of the coronavirus COVID-19 pandemic (roughly 2020 – 2022, though the virus remains present and active at the time of writing this in 2023), and it would be remiss if I didn't offer some comment based on the theories I have outlined above.

During the height of the pandemic, Germ Theory – employed by medical professionals -encouraged us to wear masks, wash our hands for a minimum of 20 seconds and maintain a distance of at least 2 metres. The belief was that by taking these steps, we could manage the microbes in order to stay healthy. A vaccination programme was also rolled out to reduce the impact of the disease.

There is, however, another side to this when we consider the questions raised around the effectiveness of wearing masks and the increase in mental health issues as a result of forced social isolation. There have been significant side effects seen in some patients who received the vaccination, including, sadly, fatalities in some who would appear to have been otherwise healthy. In addition, the lockdowns caused major disruptions for businesses, particularly hospitality, travel and education, with companies going out of business and workers being furloughed or made redundant. This (coupled with having children at home and needing to provide care and schooling) led to stress-inducing financial concerns. It is widely accepted that it will be some time before we appreciate the full impact on our health and wellbeing.

Terrain theory would guide us, in these circumstances, to address the 'health' of our terrain (surroundings, environment, etc…) and do all that we can to support this. Ways to achieve a healthier terrain could include:

- eating a healthy, unprocessed diet
- addressing any stresses in our lives – physical, emotional and/or mental

- doing all we can to live in a way that supports our True Nature, both as a species and as individuals.

Useful fact: We know from studies of animals that each species has its own optimum environmental, nutritional, social and emotional needs, and we, as humans, are no different - see the Five Freedoms of animal welfare (www.animalhumanesociety.org/health/five-freedoms-animals) which in summary states that we all need:

1. Freedom from hunger and thirst.
2. Freedom from discomfort.
3. Freedom from pain, injury or disease.
4. Freedom to express normal behaviour.
5. Freedom from fear and distress.

Good hygiene and medical advancements are, of course, important and can greatly improve our quality of life but I believe addressing our stresses, anxieties and worries while also eating a healthy diet and generally taking accountability for our wellbeing and doing all we can to support our terrain is at least as important.

As with all things, what feels right for us as an individual is a very personal choice and I'm not advocating any one particular route to follow, however I strongly recommend making our decisions consciously and with as much information and awareness as we can.

<u>Law Five</u>

Every dis-ease is part of a **natural bio-logical programme** *created to assist the organism (humans and animals alike) during unexpected distress.*

This law clearly states that dis-ease is *not* a sign of the body going wrong, making a mistake or attacking itself, but that it's an indicator of our body following our natural biological programme. Looked at this way, neither dis-ease nor microbes are things that we should fear. They are merely aspects of our body's natural wellbeing process and as such, they help us to learn and to recover our balance.

Much of the time, our best action when we start to feel unwell is to listen to our body because it's telling us – through our symptoms – what it needs. This might be rest, sleep, nutritious food or to address the stresses in our lives. However, if the UDIN has been very intense, our vitality is low, or the memory of the stressful event is repeatedly being 'retriggered', then our body can struggle to complete the process of healing. This is when we need to reach out for help, either emotional and/or medical.

What do we mean by 'retriggered'?

Essentially, this refers to the energy – the shock, stress or emotional charge - of a UDIN being reactivated. When a UDIN event occurs, our body takes a 'snapshot' of everything in its environment: sights, smells, sounds, tastes and tactile sensations. Any of these can then become associated with the stress of the UDIN, and because the body is simply trying to keep us safe, it files these things away in its cellular memory in an attempt to recognise similar threats in the future. If then, it notices these similar elements, or combinations of elements, in another situation, emotional or physical alarm bells can be triggered. Emotional alarms can cause us to feel uneasy without knowing why, whereas physical alarms can cause allergies and intolerances such as hay fever and lactose or gluten sensitivity.

If we can identify the elements (sights, smells, sounds, tastes, tactile sensations) that trigger us along with their connection to the UDIN, we will be in a position to take action and remove the unpleasant association. This will mean there is no longer any emotional charge to trigger.

To illustrate what I mean, let's take my eczema as an example. I experienced this most prominently on my eyelids and hands, areas that I felt were visible to everyone around me. I felt embarrassed and wanted to shrink away so that others didn't see my inflamed 'ugly' skin. At the same time, my inner voice was beating me up for how awful I believed I looked, all of which added to my stress. What I didn't realise at the time was that the redness, itchiness and cracked, flaky skin were actually signs that my body was trying to heal, and so, with my negative feelings producing more stress, I was actually prolonging the healing process.

> ☆ **TIP:** You might wonder if I can be so certain and, simply put, I can due to the years I have spent learning about myself and my body and applying the various tools (some of which are included in this book) to become my very own wellbeing detective. Everything I am sharing will help you to achieve the same, however, it won't necessarily be a quick fix. You will need to spend time working on all of the elements of W·I·L·D® and then using these approaches to address the issues you uncover.

In reality, the epidermis (the surface layer of our skin) is one of the tissues that thins during the Stress Phase – which is what was happening to me. This outer layer of skin relates to our sense of touch. When we experience ~

- the presence of an unwanted touch
- or the loss of a longed-for touch that is currently missing from our lives

~ then our skin thins in order to lessen this uncomfortable sensation. This can be both physical and metaphorical, and the area of the body will be significant. In the case of my hands and eyelids, these related to my desire to hold onto my relationship with my dad while at the same time being very aware that, for much of the time, I wasn't seeing him.

I have been fortunate to find and learn about Meta Consciousness®, and by employing this learning, alongside unpacking my timeline, I have become a 'wellbeing detective' and put the clues together to solve the puzzle. Yes, potentially anyone can benefit from this approach and the understanding it brings, though - as with any approach - it depends on then addressing the issues found, which sometimes we're not yet ready to do, or perhaps only to some level and not yet fully.

There aren't many clinics offering Meta Consciousness® as yet because it is not yet taught within mainstream medicine. Dr Hamer made these discoveries, but they have not been accepted by the mainstream model, which still functions under theories like Germ Theory. In fact, the medical profession classifies a very high percentage of diseases as 'idiopathic' - i.e., they have no idea why they happen or how to cure them.

Things are now changing, however, with doctors like Dr Gabor Maté and Dr Besel van der Kolk teaching about how stress can lead to disease. Others, too, are learning Dr Hamer's teachings and applying them to their work.

Theories are often dismissed initially, only to later be accepted – at which point they are then declared to be genius and ground-breaking. Changing the views of an institution like the medical profession is like changing the direction of the QE2 - it takes a lot of time and effort! If you are interested to find out more there is plenty available online - simply search for German New Medicine / Meta Medicine / Meta Health / Meta Consciousness.

Returning to my eczema and our skin's reaction, when either the missed touch is restored, or the unwanted touch is removed, or the emotional charge of the original UDIN is dissolved, the tissue feels safe to restore sensation. This allows it to regrow and heal and part of this natural process includes a stage of redness and itching. What I discovered was that each time my stress levels increased, it interrupted this healing process. And it was the body's attempt to heal that was bringing about the reappearance of my eczema symptoms.

So, though this sounds backwards, my symptoms would actually decrease when I re-entered the Stress Phase but would return tenfold when I began to relax. This is because, during this phase of relaxation, my skin was trying to heal, which meant it was entering the natural itchy, red healing process. This then caused me stress because of how I felt and how I looked, and my symptoms would decrease again. As a result, I became stuck in this recurring cycle.

Breaking the cycle only came about when I realised what the cause of my stress was – my relationship (or lack thereof) with my dad. Once I addressed my feelings around that in a way that served me better, I was able to release the trapped emotion around our lack of connection, which allowed my skin to begin to heal. When I also stopped worrying about how it looked, my skin was then able to return to normal.

Another way we can be retriggered is through our own self-talk. Again, I'll use a couple of examples from my own experience to help illustrate this.

When I was ill with ME, I used to fret about my lack of energy. It was often the focus of my thoughts, going round and around in my head how tired I was, how my muscles and joints ached and how I had no energy. At the time, I had no idea that these negative thoughts were actually contributing to and perpetuating the symptoms. What I didn't realise was that our thoughts help to create our experiences – both in ways that uplift us and in ways that bring us down. If, therefore, we feel that we're not strong, or able enough, or are 'less' in some way, and our self-talk reflects this, then it is understandable that the impact will be felt by our muscular-skeletal system, which weakens in response.

Through my learning of Meta Consciousness® and the 5 Biological Laws of Nature, I began to understand that the tissues of our muscular-skeletal system are thinned and weakened during the Stress Phase (when we are experiencing a shock or worry around our self-worth or our strength or ability to do something), so it follows that the more I worried about my lack of energy, the less energy and strength I had.

Eventually, I realised that, in order to experience full and lasting healing, it was important to focus on the good things, such as gratitude, joy, and fun and remember all the amazing things that my body had once been able to do for me. I practised focusing on these positive experiences and their uplifting physical and emotional memories and making them real again, even if only – initially - in my imagination, and finally, this led to a positive and deeper healing experience.

One of the biggest areas of (negative) self-talk in our society often surrounds the issue of weight, yet there are a number of sound biological reasons why our bodies hold the weight that doesn't in any way relate to a lack of willpower or effort on the part of the person. If we are not aware of these other factors and we try to lose weight through exercise, diet and calorie counting AND we are unsuccessful, this almost certainly leads to negative self-talk, which adds to the issue.

If weight is causing you to feel negative, it's important to take these factors into consideration:

- Consider why the body is holding the weight in the first place
- It could be water retention rather than fat, which is causing that bloated feeling and weight gain.
- Feeling judged by society for how we look can in itself be a UDIN or the reactivation of a previous UDIN, which may lead to depression. At this point, we find ourselves reaching for those highly processed 'comfort' foods, which results in further self-loathing, weight gain and a continuation of this pattern of behaviour.
- We might be under a lot of stress, which in itself leads to higher cortisol levels. Higher cortisol levels cause us to hold weight, particularly around the belly area in that 'spare tyre'.
- Cortisol also impacts our leptin levels, the hormone that lets us know when we're full. Without this, we don't know when to stop eating, and so, again, this creates a continuing cycle of behaviour. (See the diagram below.)

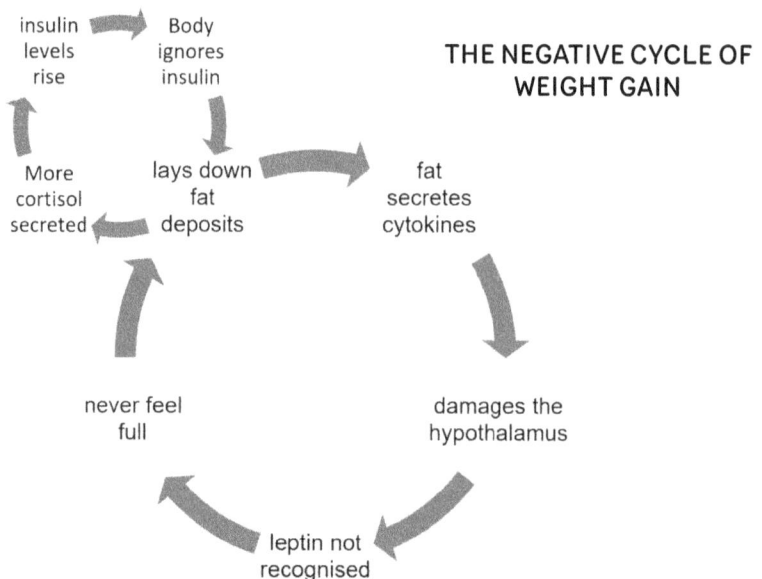

insulin levels rise → Body ignores insulin

Body ignores insulin → lays down fat deposits

lays down fat deposits → fat secretes cytokines

fat secretes cytokines → damages the hypothalamus

damages the hypothalamus → leptin not recognised

leptin not recognised → never feel full

never feel full → lays down fat deposits

lays down fat deposits → More cortisol secreted

More cortisol secreted → insulin levels rise

THE NEGATIVE CYCLE OF WEIGHT GAIN

I believe strongly that health should not be about blaming or shaming - either overtly or covertly – especially since blame and shame take away our sense of safety (see Chapter 3 for a refresher). It's not about fault. Feeling guilty or ashamed only makes things worse and perpetuates unhelpful cycles. Meta Consciousness® teaches us that it's not about 'fault' but rather about uncovering the underlying stress(es) in order to address these and free ourselves from those unhelpful cycles.

Final Note on UDIN's

It's also worth noting that we can experience additional UDINs on top of the first one, meaning we have several running concurrently. One way in which this can happen is a phenomenon known as 'diagnostic shock', which occurs when a medical diagnosis is itself a UDIN for us. That is, we find it to be Unexpected, Dramatic, and Isolating, and have No coping strategy to help us deal with it.

Taking this a step further, receiving a prognosis (positive or negative) can even create a set of beliefs which then determine the course of the dis-ease. When someone is told that they have a life-changing illness, it can have a profound impact on them. For example, let's consider a diagnosis of Multiple Sclerosis (MS). This affects the muscles which relate to a sense of not being strong, able or worthy enough to do something (UDIN 1). Receiving a diagnosis of MS and being told that they'll probably end up in a wheelchair (UDIN 2), will bring an additional fear of further deterioration in their ability to move and function. This compounds the original issue since it, too, relates to the person's sense of strength, ability and self-worth. Might it then be this second UDIN, compounding the person's sense of shock and fear, which is, in fact, the root cause of the progression of their dis-ease, turning it into a downward, self-fulfilling spiral?

It is my opinion, based on my own experience and extensive research, that everything boils down to our body awareness – the knowledge of how our body interacts with its experiences and why and how to work with this knowledge, in order to support wellbeing and help us heal from dis-ease.

Chapter Summary

- We discovered how Meta Consciousness® provides a profound insight into what's happening in our body.

- How by using this as part of our understanding and practice, it can remove the fear of dis-ease.

- Learning how our body works and interacts with both internal and external experiences can aid us in decoding our symptoms to reveal the healing wisdom they hold for us.

~ Eleven ~

Supporting Our Own Wellbeing

Inside Chapter Eleven

So, the big question which I'm sure brought you to this book was: How can I better support my own wellbeing? Having laid the groundwork for this in previous chapters, I'll now share more of the insights I've gained from my own journey. My hope is that you will find inspiration here, which will support you in developing your own Wellbeing Toolkit. Feel free to play with the ideas and practices I share and to make them uniquely your own. This is not meant to be a 'One Size Fits All' - I am simply making suggestions for you to adopt and adapt as part of your unique journey.

~ ~ ~ ~ ~

As I alluded to in the previous chapter, for me, Meta Consciousness® brings everything together.

It is about our bodies and self-awareness - knowledge of how our body interacts with its experiences and why and how we can work with this in order to support our wellbeing and help us heal from dis-ease.

I believe that much of this comes from supporting our Terrain and listening to the wisdom of our body, so throughout this chapter, I will expand on the Terrain Theory (as opposed to the Germ Theory).

I have realised that if we can find out what makes us feel:

- lighter
- free-er
- happier
- more empowered
- more at ease and comfortable within our own skin

then we can bring more of this into our lives, which is why I'm such an advocate for 'play' and 'fun'.

If we refer back to the 5 Biological Laws, we know that the thing which most upsets the balance of our Terrain is the UDIN – anything that was unexpected and dramatic for us, which felt isolating and for which we had no coping strategy. An early UDIN for me was when my dad told us that he was leaving and that my brother was Mum's favourite. This ticked all the UDIN boxes. It was Unexpected, Dramatic, Isolating, and I had No coping strategy.

We also know that this UDIN impacts our heart, brain and body and we make an adaptation (to our body) in that moment in order to survive.

This adaptation is not a conscious choice.

We don't think about it and decide to change something; we just do it. It's pure survival based on instinct. Yet, because it's so instantaneous and unconscious, it means we haven't yet processed the incident; we have simply reacted. The downside of this reaction is that the impact (of the UDIN) is still held within our body because we haven't yet received the learning it has to share with us, allowing us to release it. It is this which can lead to dis-ease.

You might wonder why, if UDINs are so harmful, our body holds onto them in this way.

Well, it isn't for masochistic reasons; quite the opposite.

Our body stores them in the hope that, at some future time, we'll be able to unpack them and benefit from their wisdom.

Just as A H Almaas explains:

> "Your conflicts, all the difficult things, the problematic situations in your life are not chance or haphazard, they're actually yours. They're specifically yours, designed specifically for you, by the part of you that loves you more than anything else. The part of you that loves you more than anything else has created roadblocks to lead you to yourself. You're not going to go in the right direction unless there's something pricking you in the side telling you, look here, this way. That part of you loves you so much that it won't let you lose the chance. It will go to extreme measures to wake you up. It will make you suffer greatly if you don't listen. What else can it do? That's its purpose."

How, then, can we benefit from the potential wisdom held within our UDINs?

It comes back to listening. We need to explore our symptoms along with their purpose or function and ask in what ways they have served us. How did they help us survive? It is easier to do this if you remember we are simply animals, like every other mammal on the planet, with basic emotions, needs and drives.

Mainstream medicine, operating based on Germ Theory, focuses on our symptoms and how to get rid of them, and it is because we are trying to get rid of them that we start to see these symptoms as unwanted and something to be avoided at all costs. This automatically takes us to a negative mindset. We will also take drugs to suppress our symptoms and use inoculations in an attempt to prevent or minimise them, again giving us the message that these symptoms are 'bad' and we need to eliminate them.

The question then is this: Does filling our bodies with these chemicals create a healthy environment?

This is not a simple question and is a complex argument, but it is worth taking a moment to consider.

There is an alternative - Salutogenesis

An alternative model, known as Salutogenesis, has been proposed, which looks at dis-ease from a different perspective. It starts with exploring what makes/keeps us well, instead of focusing on the signs of dis-ease and how to get rid of them.

Salutogenesis digs deeper into the indicators of health and wellbeing and considers how these can be enhanced or optimised. Factors that improve our health and wellbeing are referred to as 'salutogens', hence the term Salutogenesis.

Focusing on positive indicators (of wellbeing) as opposed to negative symptoms (of dis-ease) may feel like a subtle difference, but wellbeing is about so much more than just the lack of symptoms. I invite you to take a moment to sit with this idea and engage with the following exercise:

◆ Exercise: Exploring Salutogenesis

Take a piece of paper and divide it into two columns. On one side, put the heading 'Focusing on symptoms' and on the other, write 'Focusing on uplifting factors'.

In the first column, write a description or list of the (negative) symptoms you're currently experiencing. Think of all the things you've done to address these symptoms in an effort to get well. Sit for a few moments and feel into this.

In the second column, write a description or list of what your life would look like if you were able to do all the things you enjoy. Focus on the things that light you up and help you to feel good about You. Again, sit for a few moments and feel into this.

As you fill in each column, notice the emotions and sensations that come up for you. Which perspective feels more healing and opens up a greater sense of hope and potential?

> ☆ **REMEMBER:** Our thoughts create our beliefs which create our filters which determine our experiences. Phew! When you grasp this concept, you will see how much difference there truly is between these two ways of looking at health.
>
> Our thoughts ➝ Create our beliefs ➝ Create our filters

What are Salutogens?

You might be wondering what Salutogens are, and it's important to note that these positive indicators of wellbeing will vary from person to person.

I'll say that again for clarity. **Salutogens are individual and unique to each of us.**

For me, I love getting out in Nature, being around animals and spending time with family and friends. All of these activities fill me with a sense of relaxation, joy and wellbeing, so these are my salutogens.

◆ **Exercise: Pondering Salutogens**

Why not take a few moments to consider what your salutogens might be?

Make a note of at least five of them, then beside each one, add suggestion as to how you could make more time in your life to enjoy these moments (salutogens).

Types of Salutogen – Going Deeper

There are, in my experience, three 'common' salutogens – Nutrition, Movement and Self-Care. Addressing these often has a huge impact on the people who come to me.

So that you can get the most benefit from your salutogens, I have added some clarity and thoughts around each of these common types below. If you have identified salutogens that don't fall into these three categories, then it can be helpful to spend a few moments expanding on those in the same way as I have here.

- **Nutrition** – 'Diet' is a '4-letter' word for so many - I therefore like to focus instead on making sure we're getting as many nutrients as possible (and avoid using the word 'diet').

  The saying 'eat the rainbow' is actually valid because each colour we eat offers us a different set of vitamins and minerals. Eating slowly and mindfully and doing your best to avoid highly processed foods where possible is also really beneficial. Alongside this, it is important to keep well-hydrated.

  If you have any concerns about your diet, you can ask a kinesiologist to check your system to see if you lack any nutrients. They will also be able to identify what foods and/or supplements will help you to address this[1]. If any lack is found, it's worth exploring whether there might be issues which are making it difficult for your body to absorb these nutrients and potentially seek medical advice as well.

  In addition, when I think of nourishing and nurturing (nutrition), I consider everything that we 'take in' – not just what we eat – such as:

  - ? what we listen to – including TV, radio, podcasts, general everyday conversations, and our self-talk
  - ? what we read – including social media posts, newspapers and books.

  Think about whether these lift you up or weigh you down – or maybe they even wind you up. Remember that we get to choose.

---

1 *A note about supplements – bear in mind that though these can be hugely beneficial, they can be expensive, particularly if you need to take them for any length of time. It can be worth doing your own research to find the most appropriate solution for you.*

If you feel you can't avoid something or someone that's bringing you down or making you anxious, then make a mental note to take some self-care action later. This will enable you to offload any unhelpful energy at the earliest opportunity.

TIP: Make sure you follow through on this action because that will show your body that you're actively listening and taking steps to address the issues it shares with you. Your body will then no longer feel it needs to shout (leading to intense symptoms) and you will be able to develop a more effective dialogue and understanding.

- **Movement** – Exercise can often be something that we feel we 'have to' do, and sometimes we even use it to 'punish' ourselves. Have you, for example, ever tried to work out how many calories you've consumed and then how many hours of exercise it would take to burn these off? Whilst this activity is undoubtedly 'movement', it is coming from a place of negative bias, so instead, why not think of movement as a way to celebrate all the wonderful things your body can do for you? Think about what forms of movement you enjoy. Like Dancing!

Wouldn't that be so much more fun?

- **Self-care** – Stress has developed a bit of a bad reputation in society, yet a certain amount of it is necessary. In fact, it's the stress hormones adrenaline and cortisol that help us to get out of bed in the morning. They are the ones motivating us and providing the energy to achieve our goals. Instead of thinking about stress as 'bad' then, what if we looked at how we could develop a robust and regular self-care practice (to offset our stress), one that enabled us to feel safe and comfortable, to be ourselves, and to take time out for the things we enjoy?

Your self-care practice could include things such as massages and spending time in Nature, but to be truly effective, it's also important to make time to explore and address the areas of disconnection, pain, shame and 'shadow' that we carry within us.

> **TIP:** A good place to start your self-care practice is to visit the Self-Care Exercises playlist on my YouTube channel (https://equenergy.com/SelfCareExercises). There you'll find videos sharing simple exercises you can use to explore both your physical sensations and your emotional feelings, and how to support and nurture yourself through this process.

Another very important aspect of self-care is making sure that we get sufficient quality rest and sleep. By rest, I mean taking time in silence and stillness. This can be through meditation, mindfulness, or just sitting quietly and giving ourselves the space and time to listen to our own inner voice of wisdom. Many of us live in such a busy, noisy world that making time for silence and stillness can be challenging. It can feel rather alien initially, too, so consider what would support you in getting started.

> **TIP:** If you'd like to have a deeper understanding of why sleep is so vital to our wellbeing, take a look at Matthew Walker's 'eye-opening' book, "*Why We Sleep: The New Science of Sleep and Dreams.*"

Remember - be compassionate towards that part of you which might feel restless and/or frustrated. It's well worth persisting with this practice because I know from my own experience how big a role it plays in helping us reconnect with those parts of ourselves from which we have become disconnected.

When we decide to take our self-care seriously and do whatever it takes to support our wellbeing, we can use our previous personal experiences as guides.

Using previous personal experiences as guides

To do this, review these experiences (during or following on from any situation which brings up an emotional or physical reaction) and then ask some of the following questions:

- How did I feel about what happened?

  Not what did others feel, or what 'should' I have felt, but how did I ACTUALLY FEEL?

  It's about focusing on your emotions at this point – your feelings – instead of thinking about why we think things happened the way they did. Our sense of 'why' is an interpretation, our perception and is not helpful at this point.

- What impact did the event have on me?

  Explore how you felt after the event and whether your thoughts, beliefs, approach or behaviour changed because of what happened.

- What meaning did I give to what happened?

  Having got clear on your answers to the above questions, you can now focus on your interpretation – your perception - of events. As you have already figured out how you really felt, you now have a solid foundation on which to challenge your perception.

- What beliefs did I create about myself in that moment?

  Or if this is a situation that you've found yourself in before, ask yourself: What beliefs was I holding about myself during the event?

  Events which we find upsetting can leave us feeling small and vulnerable, even powerless – and we know that powerless is right down at the bottom of the Emotion Scale (to see the diagram again, go to Appendix 1). And this was where I felt myself to be before starting my search for healing.

It's easy for me to say, though, for I have discovered my healing and am sharing these learnings with you from a positive place – but if you're feeling powerless, how can you start to make that change? In a nutshell – **by taking back your responsibility.**

I'd like to clarify here that I'm not saying, 'take responsibility' in the sense of 'you brought this on yourself; you sort it out'.

Similarly, I don't mean taking responsibility for everything and everyone and worrying about the slightest little thing that might upset others. The only person you can impact is yourself, so I have learned that worrying about others simply doesn't serve me. Me worrying didn't help the people around me; it didn't help the people and situations reported in the news, and it certainly didn't help me! (I'm also not suggesting that we shouldn't care or take action to support others, just that the worry and anxiety it can cause are often unhelpful and can be detrimental to our own health).

What I came to understand was that **I was assuming responsibility for things which weren't mine to worry about**, and this was a huge realisation. A lightbulb moment if you like, and a real turning point.

When I realised I was taking on responsibility that was not mine to take, I was able to explore why I'd taken this on and make any adjustments as appropriate. It can be helpful here to think of the things in our lives that we have a degree of control over, the areas where we have a greater or lesser degree of influence and the things which are outside of our control – although these may still impact us.

◆ Exercise: Explore your own Circles of Control

Take ten minutes to draw these circles on a piece of paper and have a go at filling them in for your current situation. You'll be surprised at how many things you are worrying about that you have no influence or control over whatsoever. Once you've done this, it's easy to see which you can eliminate from your responsibility.

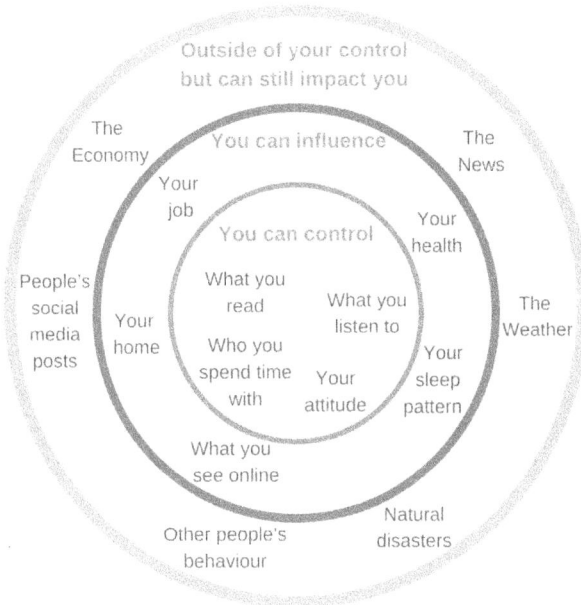

THE CIRCLES OF CONTROL

Learning what areas *are your responsibility* is the first step towards a journey of self-care.

Of course, self-care is not always possible in the exact moment - as any fraught parent or tired caregiver will tell you – but when it is possible to make time for self-care, it's important to make it a priority or, to put it another way, a conscious choice. Remember, we have that choice, and it is so important that we look after ourselves, particularly if we are responsible for the care of others.

Responsibility and self-care

I started talking about 'responsibility' as a way to begin your self-care journey and to address any feelings of powerlessness. In this sense, appropriate responsibility could also be called response-ability, that is, our ability to respond rather than just react. When we respond as opposed to react, when we consciously choose what to say or how to behave in a situation, it is incredibly empowering. How many times have you reacted to a situation only to regret your actions later?

So, becoming response-able for our choices – consciously taking a moment of pause to choose our response whilst also taking accountability for any consequences - gives us back our sense of agency (control). We no longer feel powerless and learn so much more about ourselves in the process.

It's not always an easy journey – it requires us to take a very honest look at ourselves and come face-to-face with our 'shadow' - but if we can remember that our shadow is just a part of ourselves which is feeling unloved, unwanted and rejected, we can see the value it has to offer us. We looked at this in a bit more detail at the end of Chapter 7, where we discussed gently embracing this aspect of ourselves and working with it rather than trying to fight against it. Believe me, the end result is worth it.

One final point I'd like to make, in relation to radical self-care, is about the concept of acceptance and what acceptance is NOT.

Acceptance is NOT saying things like, "I guess I'll just have to accept things and move on," because you won't be addressing the underlying issue. Attempting to 'push down' your pain in the hope that it will go away does not work and can lead to resentment. The pain remains in your body, ready to burst out again at a later date – like a squeezed stress ball – and will emerge when you experience another trigger that reignites the energy of the original UDIN.

It is my opinion that the whole healing journey is about true acceptance: about finding peace with whatever the issue might be and then addressing the resulting feelings with honesty. This is not easy, and I would never pretend otherwise, but if we face our issues with honesty, curiosity, and, crucially, also with deep compassion, then we can make a change.

If we make space for our discomforts and our fears and invite them to teach us more about ourselves - while staying open and continuing to practice deep Self-Love – we can learn how to hold that compassionate space for ourselves.

And, once we can do this, in my experience, this is where we find true and lasting healing.

Chapter Summary

- We looked at how we can best support our wellbeing.

- We took a deeper dive into the differences between Terrain Theory and Germ Theory, exploring how they influence our perspectives on dis-ease.

- We also learned about the concept of Radical Self-Care and how this can be achieved.

- We reminded ourselves that our practices should always be gentle and involve the element of fun.

~ Twelve ~

Conclusion

Inside Chapter Twelve

You are the expert in your own body, experiences, and situation. No one else has walked in your shoes.

~ ~ ~ ~ ~

I want to make it clear that I'm not saying mainstream medicine is 'bad' or 'wrong' and should be avoided. On the contrary, doctors, hospitals and medications have important roles to play in our health.

Meta Consciousness® and my W·I·L·D® strategy, are both very much complementary approaches that seek to work alongside medical professionals in a partnership where both sides come together for the benefit of the person they're supporting. Personally, I believe in empowering others to make the most informed choices they possibly can and to follow the path that's right for them as individuals, which is how I seek to support my clients.

It is crucial that people have the confidence to talk to any practitioner and to ask the questions that will assist them in making their decisions and that the practitioner will listen and respond appropriately. After all, we are the experts on our bodies and know the most about the experiences we have encountered, especially around dis-ease.

> **TIP:** Whoever you approach for support, make sure you are able to retain your sense of agency and control over your own wellbeing. There is nothing more powerful than simply being YOU when it comes to your healing toolkit.

If there's one thing I'd like to achieve with this book, it's to start reducing the fears that so many of us carry. Some fears, of course, are natural, normal and even healthy – these are the ones that help to keep us safe, such as the fear of heights or of fire. But there are other fears – the ones that have come from the traumas (UDINs) we've experienced – which leave us in some way 'less' than we were before.

According to Gabor Maté (from *The Myth of Normal: Trauma, Illness & Healing in a Toxic Culture*) these fears (if unaddressed) can result in:

- a limitation/constriction/diminishing of capacity to feel/think/trust yourself.
- having less capacity to assert yourself or to experience suffering without succumbing to despair.
- a reduced capacity to witness suffering with compassion.
- holding on to your pain, sorrow and fear.
- feeling overwhelmed.
- using busy-ness, overworking and other 'escapist'/addictive behaviours.
- having a compulsive need for self-soothing/self-stimulating, by whatever means.
- feeling compelled to either puff up/hide in order to 'fit in' /find acceptance/justify your existence.
- impairment of your capacity to experience gratitude for the beauty and wonder of life.
- feeling restricted, constricted, or narrowed in some way, with decreased emotional resilience and flexibility.

One way that we can start to reduce our fears is to be kind to ourselves, and through this book, I'd like to help you gain a sense of yourself as a truly wonder-full and beauty-full being.

I also hope you will understand that you are doing the best you can with the resources you have available to you at this moment and that it's okay to take the pressure off and give yourself permission for self-care and exploration. In addition, I hope you will start to make more time for fun and not take life so seriously – which is a big one for me.

Why?

Because we only get this one time here in this human body, having this particular human adventure, and so the Life we are experiencing is about living every moment to the full, extracting every nuance of experience and enjoying (in-joying) it as much as we possibly can.

With this in mind, I'd like to share something that I wrote for a collaborative book project (Words of the Wise[2]) a while ago. It's in the form of a letter, written from the perspective of Who We Really Are to our Human Self:

Dearest One

I wanted to reach out to you to say that I've seen the challenges you've been facing and all that you've been doing to navigate through the sometimes stormy seas. I've watched you question yourself, wondering whether you have what it takes, whether you're making the right choices and, at times, if you'll ever make it through to calmer waters.

I know that at times you've felt disorientated, lost and alone, even losing sight of the wonder of Who You Really Are and the amazing gifts you bring. So, I wanted to let you know you are not alone. I am here, right by your side, all along the way.

When times feel hard, I'm there supporting you.
When times feel good, I'm there celebrating with you.
When you feel that you're the only one on this path, just look up, and you'll see me there cheering you on.

You might not be able to see me with your eyes, but you will know and recognise me from your heart. I'm there in the little things:

*   *the sun after the clouds*

---

2   You can find the book of this title on Amazon at https://equenergy.com/WordsOfTheWise

* the refreshing rain at the end of a long, hot day
* the smile of a child
* the purr of a cat
* the wag of a dog's tail
* a breeze through the leaves of a tree as it gently caresses your skin
* the phone call or e-mail from a friend
* the ocean
* the sunrise and sunset
* the moon and the stars.

In all of these things, I send my love to you. I long to fill you and surround you with this love and for it to empower you and connect you with all the wisdom and resources carried within you. But sometimes I see things weighing you down and blinding you to my love. And so, I'm writing to tell you directly how special, how precious you are to me.

I created you over many generations, carefully selecting the very particular aspects of being that went into forming such a wanted and treasured child, both the things that you have labelled 'good' and the things that you or others have called 'unwanted' or 'undesirable'. To me, they are all just aspects of my beloved child. Both 'good' and 'undesirable' have their strengths and weaknesses, but when they come together in the love I wish to share with you, then their true beauty, power and majesty shine for all to see. Then love, light, and joy shine from you unto all around you and light up the world with that love.

Please take these words to your heart, dear one. Release your worries and fears and your need to take life so seriously. Relax into the knowledge of my love and the safe space in which you are so gently held.

Life is not a test. You can't 'get it wrong' or 'fail'. If things don't work out the way you'd hoped, just smile, call out "Plot

twist", and start over. I'll be right there laughing along with
you and cheering you every step of the way. And if you ever need
to feel my presence, to feel my arms around you and to know the
truth of all that I've shared, just find a place of stillness, close
your eyes and gently reach out with your heart. I'll be there.

Yours always – forever.

Your Soul Self [3]

As we continue on this wonderful journey of life, it's normal for us to become concerned about many things, not least of which is the fear of dis-ease. I hope, that I have been able to show you how natural dis-ease is and that it has a purpose in supporting our learning and growth. The challenges we can experience through dis-ease are simply landmarks on the road map to our True Nature.

Remember: Dis-ease is not a sign of weakness, and it's not our 'fault'. It's actually a sign that our body is trying to process and release some kind of stress. The toxins it produces as a by-product of this stress are what result in our symptoms. When we understand this and can make space for the body to complete its healing process, it brings us a greater sense of self-awareness and calm.

Author Note: When a condition has become chronic, this is an indication that something of the original trauma has not yet been released, and so it is still active in our body. Over time, this can potentially lead to life-limiting conditions and perhaps a terminal diagnosis, but even in these situations, it is possible to take action to support greater wellbeing. According to *Terminal Cancer is a Misdiagnosis* by Danny Carroll and *Radical Remission* by Kelly A Turner - given the right conditions, healing can still be achieved.

There are lots of techniques we can use to support ourselves; it's about finding the ones that work best for you.

---

3   *This is also available as a video on my YouTube channel at https://equenergy.com/letter*

(Bear in mind that these techniques vary over time and from situation to situation, so it's good to keep an open mind and try out a variety of different approaches. It can be useful to keep a record of the things you have tried and the outcome so that you can discover which techniques are more beneficial to you).

Personally, I've explored several, including:

- massage and reflexology
- movement
- music
- drawing
- singing
- gong baths – 'bathing' in sound vibrations can help to put us into a meditative, healing state
- meditation
- mindfulness
- hypnotherapy
- homeopathy
- essential oils
- Bach Flower Remedies – very gentle, uplifting essences used to support emotional release and healing[4]
- Reiki[5] / Energy Healing and other energy-based practices
- Shiatsu, Amatsu (beautiful, gentle, Japanese soft-tissue therapies) [6]
- Yoga, Qi Gong and Tai Chi offer mindful movement to support us in becoming more aware of and comfortable within our own bodies
- acupuncture and acupressure
- breathing exercises

---

4   *For further information see https://www.bachcentre.com/en/remedies/*
5   *Rei Ki means 'Life-Force Energy'. The Reiki practitioner gets into the higher vibrational states of Love and Gratitude and then offers this to the person they're working with in order for them to experience the inner sense of peace and acceptance that enables healing.*
6   *For further information see https://www.amatsutherapyintl.com/what-is-amatsu.html*

⇨ grounding exercises

⇨ nutrition

⇨ Emotional Freedom Technique (EFT) – also known as 'tapping' - helps us to release emotions which have been causing pain and discomfort

⇨ Matrix Reimprinting (MR) – a particular way of using EFT that helps to address past trauma and create positive beliefs for the future

⇨ and, of course, Nature.

This list is far from exhaustive, and you may well find others which resonate with you more. Any approach or technique is a very personal choice, so it's worth exploring those that you feel drawn to and discover which ones work for you.

In my work (and daily life), the ones I draw on most often are EFT, MR and Reiki, along with other energy-based practices such as breathing, grounding, guided meditations and exploring Nature. I bring these into my 1:1 sessions and workshops, and they also feed into my Create Your own W·I·L·D® Wellbeing learning programme. If you'd like to learn more about any of these and discover how they might support you in creating the life that you long to live, then please get in touch. You can find all my details by scanning the QR code in Appendix 2 or going to my website: *www.equenergy.com*

In summary, living a W·I·L·D® life is about BE-ing rather than DO-ing. It's about:

√ giving yourself permission to be faithful to your True Nature.

√ embracing the **Wonder** of Life, even when it feels messy, uncertain and uncomfortable.

√ trusting your **Intuition**.

√ learning to **Love** all of who you are and to fully embrace this – the 'light'* and the 'shadow'.

√ learning how to **Dance** with Life – to trust that Life is on your side, wanting you to thrive and to fully experience as much joy-full living as you can.

It's also about how you do whatever you choose to do, rather than what you choose to do. It's not a competition. Life isn't judging you; you can't get it 'wrong', and you can't 'fail'. It's just about being as You as you possibly can – and who better to do that than you?!

So, go on – give yourself permission to enjoy (in-joy) this thing called Life. Don't take it too seriously. Make time for you and time for fun. Follow your heart and allow space for the things that light you up and make your heart sing.

And if you're finding this challenging right now – perhaps you're reading this book and thinking, 'Where on Earth do I start? How do I do this?', or possibly even 'I can't do this, I haven't got what it takes' – then reach out to someone you trust, whether that be a friend, a family member or a professional practitioner. You don't have to do this alone. There's absolutely no shame in asking for some support. Remember, this is your journey - you get to call the shots and make the decisions and choices that are right for you. You do not have to do anything simply to please others. Their suggestions and advice might be sound – but perhaps only for them because no one else knows what it's like to walk in your shoes.

So, trust your body, listen to that in-tuition and do what you feel is right for you. And if it doesn't work out as well as you'd hoped, that's fine; you're perfectly free to make a new choice and go in a completely different direction.

I wish you all the very best with your ongoing adventures as you start out on your own personal Walk on the W·I·L·D® Side.

* Marianne Williamson wrote a beautiful poem about our light which had a profound impact on me and I refer back to it often:

Our Deepest Fear

By Marianne Williamson

Our deepest fear is not that we are inadequate.
Our deepest fear is that we are powerful beyond measure.
It is our light, not our darkness
That most frightens us.
We ask ourselves
Who am I to be brilliant, gorgeous, talented, fabulous?
Actually, who are you not to be?
You are a child of God.
You're playing small
Does not serve the world.
There's nothing enlightened about shrinking
So that other people won't feel insecure around you.
We are all meant to shine,
As children do.
We were born to make manifest
The glory of God that is within us.
It's not just in some of us;
It's in everyone.
And as we let our own light shine,
We unconsciously give other people permission to do the same.
As we're liberated from our own fear,
Our presence automatically liberates others.

This inspiring poem is taken from Marianne Williamson's book *A Return to Love*.

A Closing Note from Robyn

Hey there,

First of all I'd like to say a massive THANK YOU for taking this bold step and diving into "Take a Walk on the W·I·L·D® Side". It warms my heart to know you're part of this journey.

Being on the healing path is a profound adventure and having you along for the ride is an absolute honour. Your thoughts on the book mean the world to me. Whether it's a quick email (_robyn@equenergy.com_), a cosy Zoom chat (_https://equenergy.com/bookachat_), or a few kind words on Amazon, I'm all ears and truly appreciate your feedback.

Let's keep the connection alive! Follow me on LinkedIn, Facebook, Instagram, and YouTube – all the links can be found in the business e-card in Appendix 7.

There's a buzzing private space on Facebook too, our _Walking On The W·I·L·D® Side_ group at _www.facebook.com/groups/walkingonthewildside_. Join us for some extra warmth and wisdom. Pop your email in during the group questions - I promise no spam, and I'll never share details. This signs you up to receive my W·I·L·D® Way guide, filled with extra self-care treasures and tools. You'll also get a monthly dose of insights and my quarterly newsletter, W·I·L·D® Times. You're in control, and you can unsubscribe at any time.

Your journey doesn't end with the last page—it's just beginning.

Wishing you a fantastic journey ahead in all your wellbeing adventures.

You've got this!

With W·I·L·D® love,

Robyn ♥

APPENDICES

Appendix 1: The Emotion Scale

Appendix 2: Safety

Appendix 3: Cook's Hook Up Exercise

Appendix 4: Values List

Appendix 5: Hakalau

Appendix 6: The Emotion Wheel

Appendix 7: Contact Me

Appendix 1: The Emotion Scale

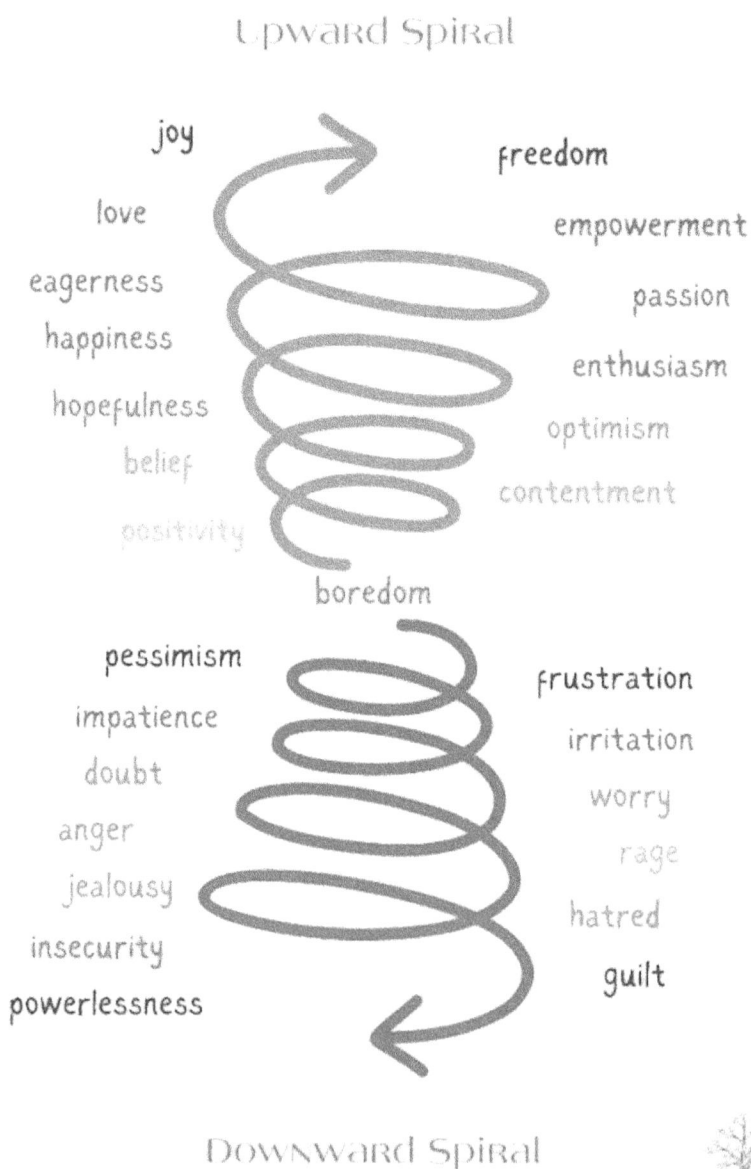

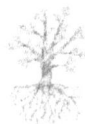

Upward Spiral

joy

freedom

love

empowerment

eagerness

passion

happiness

enthusiasm

hopefulness

optimism

belief

contentment

positivity

boredom

pessimism

frustration

impatience

irritation

doubt

worry

anger

rage

jealousy

hatred

insecurity

guilt

powerlessness

Downward Spiral

Appendix 2: Safety

SAFETY

this is such an important concept for
our healing and ongoing wellbeing,
but what does it actually mean?

Well, for me it's:

that we
feel **Safe**

enough
to be our **Authentic**
self

knowing we
have the **Freedom**

to **Express**

our **True Nature**

- ie for you
to be fully **You** ☆

without fear of judgment or loss of
attachment / connection

© EQUENERGY.COM

Appendix 3: Cook's Hook Up

This is a great little exercise if you're feeling 'out of sorts' or you're having one of those days where you're experiencing clumsy-ness or clunky-ness. You know, when you can't seem to string a sentence together!

1. Start by doing the 'clap' test to find out which is your dominant side (this might not be the same as whether you're right or left-handed so bear with me). Imagine you've just seen your favourite band at a live gig, or a fabulous play at the theatre and you start to clap in appreciation. Now, notice which hand is on top, or which hand is doing most of the movement. This is your dominant hand.

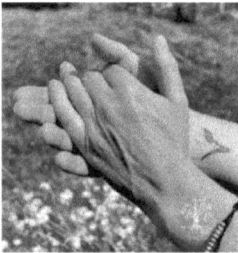

2. Next, sit down and stretch both arms straight out in front of you, at right angles to your body.

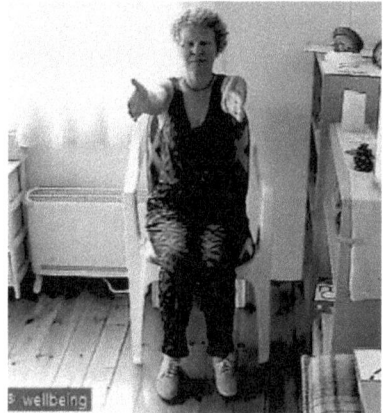

3. Now cross your dominant arm over your other arm and then twist it around so that your palms are facing each other.

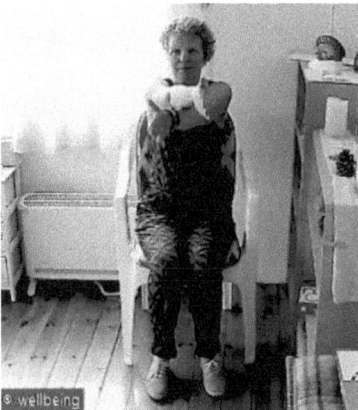

4. Interlace your fingers and then bring your interlocked hands under and up so that they're in contact with your chest - just above your heart.

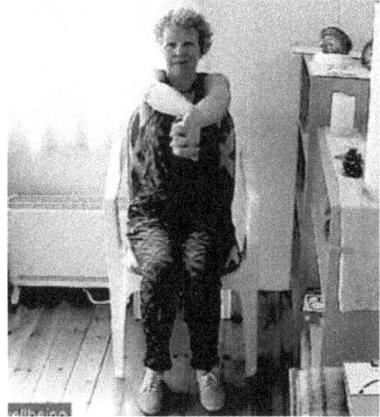

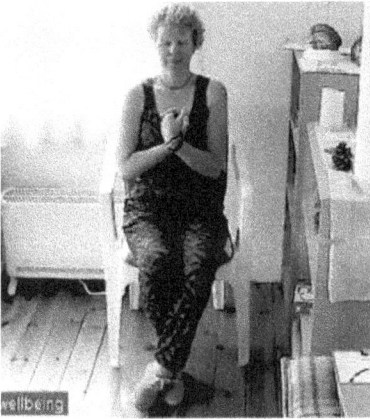

5. Now, cross your non-dominant ankle over your other ankle.

6. Say the following phrase out loud to yourself, three times:

   "Right here, right now, in this moment, I am safe."

7. Repeat this quietly to yourself until you feel some kind of physical, emotional or spiritual shift within your body. When you feel this shift, you can un-cross your arms and legs.

8. Next, steeple your fingers in front of your chest and repeat the statement out loud to yourself another three times:

   "Right here, right now, in this moment, I am safe."

(image on next page)

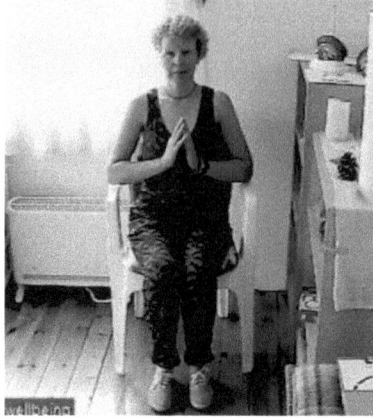

"Right here, right now, in this moment I am safe."

If you were using this exercise to prepare for the Sway Test on page 142, you can now return to it and see if this has enabled your body to sway. If it hasn't, repeat this exercise and drink some more water.

This should be sufficient for you to re-regulate your body. If not, it might be that your vitality is low, in which case you could try out some of the suggestions for boosting the wellbeing of your Terrain which were given in Chapter Ten (pg. 203 onwards).

Appendix 4: Values List

- Acceptance
- Accomplishment
- Accountability
- Accuracy
- Achievement
- Adaptability
- Adventurousness
- Agreeableness
- Alertness
- Altruism
- Ambition
- Amiability
- Amusement
- Amusingness
- Articulateness
- Assertiveness
- Athleticism
- Attentiveness
- Authenticity
- Awe
- Balance
- Beauty
- Bliss
- Boldness
- Brilliance
- Calmness
- Capability
- Carefulness
- Caring
- Cautiousness
- Certainty
- Charisma
- Charm
- Cheerfulness
- Citizenship
- Clarity
- Cleanliness
- Clear-headedness
- Cleverness
- Comfort
- Commitment
- Common sense
- Communication
- Community
- Compassion
- Competence
- Complexity
- Confidence
- Connection
- Conscientiousness
- Conservativeness
- Consideration
- Consistency
- Constructiveness
- Contemplation
- Contentment
- Contribution
- Control
- Conviction
- Cooperation
- Courage
- Courteousness
- Craftiness
- Creativity
- Credibility
- Curiosity
- Daringness
- Decency
- Decisiveness
- Dedication

- Deep thought
- Democracy
- Dependability
- Determination
- Devotion
- Dignity
- Diligence
- Discipline
- Diversity
- Drive
- Dualism
- Dutifulness
- Easygoingness
- Education
- Effectiveness
- Efficiency
- Elegance
- Eloquence
- Emotional awareness
- Emotional control
- Empathy
- Empowerment
- Endurance
- Energy
- Enjoyment
- Enthusiasm
- Equality
- Ethics
- Excellence
- Excitement
- Expedience
- Experimentation
- Exploration
- Expressiveness
- Fairness
- Faith
- Family
- Farsightedness
- Fidelity
- Flair
- Flexibility
- Focus
- Foresight
- Forgiving
- Forthrightness
- Fortitude
- Freedom
- Friendliness
- Fun
- Generosity
- Gentleness
- Good-nature
- Goodness
- Grace
- Graciousness
- Gratitude
- Greatness
- Growth
- Happiness
- Hard work
- Harmony
- Health
- Helpfulness
- Heroism
- Honesty
- Honour
- Hope
- Humility
- Humour
- Idealism
- Imagination
- Incisiveness
- Independence
- Individualism
- Individuality
- Influence

- Innovation
- Insightfulness
- Inspiration
- Integrity
- Intelligence
- Intensity
- Intuitiveness
- Inventiveness
- Joy
- Justice
- Kindness
- Knowledge
- Lawfulness
- Leadership
- Learning
- Liberty
- Likability
- Logic
- Love
- Loyalty
- Mastery
- Maturity
- Mellowness
- Moderation
- Modesty
- Motivation
- Neatness
- Neutrality
- Newness
- Niceness
- Objectivity
- Open-mindedness
- Openness
- Optimism
- Order
- Organisation
- Originality
- Passion
- Patience
- Patriotism
- Peace
- Peacefulness
- Performance
- Perseverance
- Persistence
- Playfulness
- Pleasure
- Poise
- Positive attitude
- Positivity
- Practicality
- Preciseness
- Principles
- Productivity
- Professionalism
- Prosperity
- Protection
- Punctuality
- Purpose
- Quality
- Rationality
- Realism
- Recognition
- Recreation
- Reflection
- Relaxation
- Reliability
- Resourcefulness
- Respect
- Responsibility
- Restraint
- Results-oriented
- Rigor
- Risk
- Romance
- Satisfaction

- Security
- Self-awareness
- Self-improvement
- Self-reliance
- Self-respect
- Self-sufficiency
- Selflessness
- Sensitivity
- Serenity
- Service
- Simplicity
- Sociability
- Spirituality
- Spontaneity
- Stability
- Status
- Steadiness
- Strength
- Structure
- Studiousness
- Success
- Sweetness
- Sympathy
- Tenderness
- Thoroughness
- Tidiness
- Timeliness
- Tolerance
- Tradition
- Tranquillity
- Transformation
- Trust
- Truth
- Unity
- Variety
- Vivaciousness
- Warmth
- Wealth
- Well-roundedness
- Wisdom
- Wit

Source: *berkeleywellbeing.com*

Appendix 5: Hakalau

1. Stare at a spot that's just above eye level - so that your eyes feel like they're bumping off your eyebrows.
2. Look at this spot until it goes fuzzy, a ring appears around it, or it appears to move.
3. When this happens, look away, then stare at the spot again.
4. Now, allow your focus to soften and open out so that you become aware of your peripheral vision as well as what's directly in front of you. Practice this at least **four** times a day.

The Active Meditation of the Kahuna

One meaning of Hakalau is, *"to stare at, as in meditation, and to allow to spread out."* If you've never tried it before, this technique can be a real revelation.

- **Ho'ohaka**: Just pick a spot on the wall to look at, preferably above eye level so that your field of vision seems to bump up against your eyebrows, but the eyes are not so high as to cut off the field of vision.
- **Kuu**: *"To let go."* As you stare at this spot, just let your mind go loose and focus all of your attention on the spot.
- **Lau**: *"To spread out."* Notice that within a matter of moments, your vision begins to spread out, and you see more in the peripheral than you do in the central part of your vision.
- **Hakalau**: Now, pay attention to the peripheral. In fact, pay more attention to the peripheral than to the central part of your vision.
- **Ho'okohi**: Stay in this state for as long as you can. Notice how it feels. Notice the ecstatic feelings that begin to come to you as you continue the state.

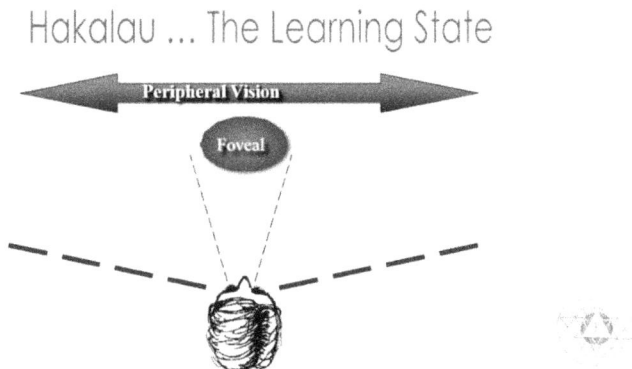

Hakalau ... The Learning State

Peripheral Vision

Foveal

251

Appendix 6: The Emotion Wheel

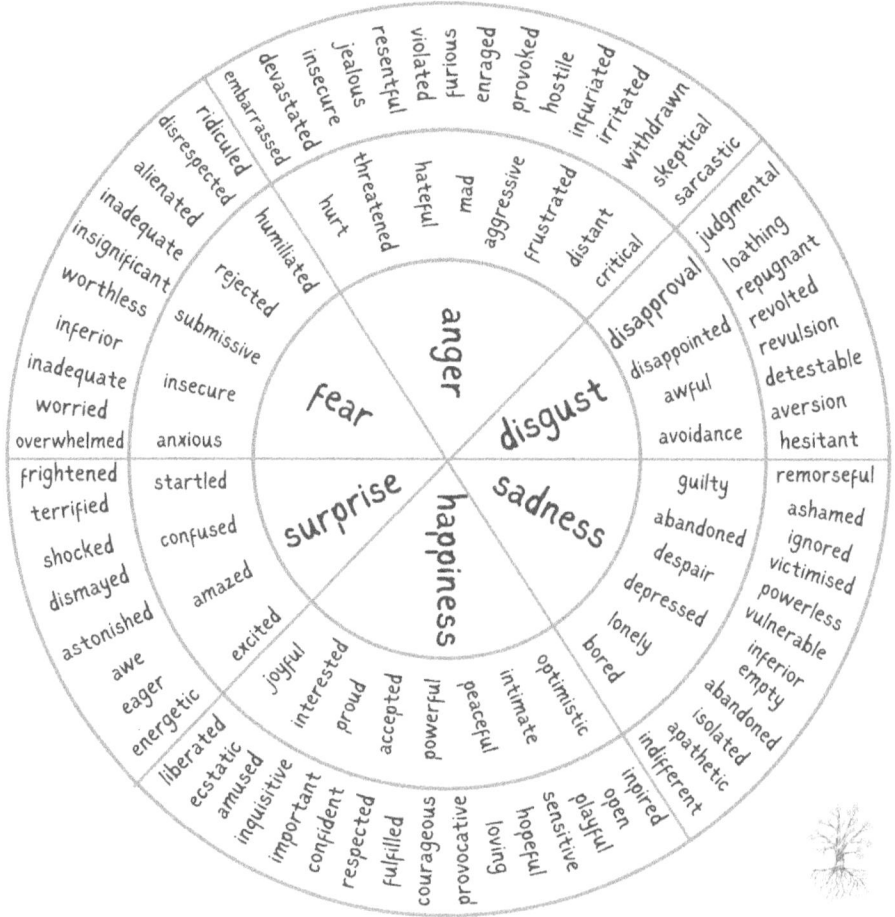

Appendix 7: Contact Me

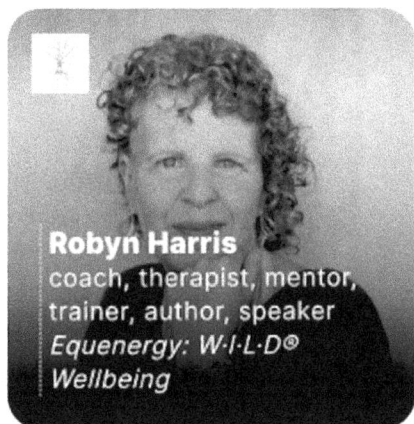

Robyn Harris
coach, therapist, mentor,
trainer, author, speaker
*Equenergy: W·I·L·D®
Wellbeing*

https://equenergy.com/BusinessCard

BOOKS AND RESOURCES

USEFUL RESOURCES

Web Links: (Alphabetical Order)

- **7 Tips for finding the practitioner who's right for you:** https://www.equenergy.com/7-tips-for-finding-the-practitioner-whos-right-for-you/

- **Abraham Hicks:** https://www.abraham-hicks.com/

- **Amatsu**: https://www.amatsutherapyintl.com/what-is-amatsu.html

- **Bach Flower Remedy information**: https://www.bachcentre.com/en/remedies/

- **Body Scan exercise:** https://equenergy.com/BodyScan/

- **Bone and joint case study:** https://learninggnm.com/SBS/documents/Alvin_Case_95_E.pdf

- **Chronic fatigue syndrome**: https://en.wikipedia.org/wiki/Chronic_fatigue_syndrome

- **Cochrane Review, January 2023**: https://www.cochranelibrary.com/cdsr/doi/10.1002/14651858.CD006207.pub6/full

- **Create Your Own W·I·L·D® Wellbeing Programme:** https://www.equenergy.com/create-your-own-wild-programme

- **Gabor Maté: How Repressed Anger Affects Your Health**: https://www.youtube.com/watch?v=KSc1GDNC4b4

- **Germ Theory versus Terrain Theory**
  - » https://www.nutritionist-resource.org.uk/memberarticles/germ-theory-vs-terrain-theory-in-relation-to-the-coronavirus
  - » https://www.westonaprice.org/health-topics/notes-from-yesteryear/germ-theory-versus-terrain-the-wrong-side-won-the-day/#gsc.tab=0

- **Giving Wellbeing Some Horse Power**: https://www.equenergy.com/GivingWellbeingSomeHorsePower

- **Health statistics**
  - » https://assets.publishing.service.gov.uk/media/60c892108fa8f57ce980b6b7/GO-Science_Trend_Deck_-_Health_Section_-_Spring_2021.pdf
  - » https://www.ons.gov.uk/peoplepopulationandcommunity/healthandsocialcare/conditionsanddiseases/bulletins/cancerregistrationstatisticsengland/2017#cancer-diagnoses-continue-to-increase
  - » www.gov.uk/government/statistics/prescription-cost-analysis-england-2016
  - » http://healthsurvey.hscic.gov.uk/media/63790/HSE2016-pres-med.pdf
  - » https://www.statista.com/statistics/418091/prescription-items-dispensed-in-england/
  - » https://www.bbc.co.uk/news/health-58639253

- **Homeostasis:** https://www.britannica.com/science/homeostasis

- **How reintroducing wolves to Yellowstone National Park changed the course of the rivers:** https://www.youtube.com/watch?v=ysa5OBhXz-Q&t=69s

- **Irritable Bowel Syndrome:** https://en.wikipedia.org/wiki/Irritable_bowel_syndrome

- **Manifesting**
  - » https://trueselfmanifestation.com/intuition-manifesting
  - » https://www.vox.com/the-goods/21524975/manifesting-does-it-really-work-meme

- **Microbes**
  - » https://www.ncbi.nlm.nih.gov/books/NBK279387/
  - » https://languages.oup.com/

- **Reiki**: www.reiki.org

- **Risks posed by microplastics:** https://www.webmd.com/a-to-z-guides/news/20221028/microplastics-health-risks-what-do-we-really-know

- **Safey and side effects of covid vaccines:** https://www.nhs.uk/conditions/covid-19/covid-19-vaccination/covid-19-vaccines-side-effects-and-safety/

- **Salutogenesis:** https://www.merriam-webster.com/dictionary/salutogenesis

- **Schizophrenia**: https://www.therecoveryvillage.com/mental-health/schizotypal-personality-disorder/

- **Self-Care Exercises:** https://equenergy.com/SelfCareExercises

- **Stress isn't all bad:** https://www.youtube.com/watch?v=RcGyVTAoXEU

- **The Adverse Childhood Experiences test:** https://developingchild.harvard.edu/media-coverage/take-the-ace-quiz-and-learn-what-it-does-and-doesnt-mean/

- **The Cerebral Cortex**: https://my.clevelandclinic.org/health/articles/23073-cerebral-cortex

- **The Focus Wheel by Abraham-Hicks:** https://www.youtube.com/watch?v=Vv_DBfgLhjM

- **Trauma is a 'stupid friend' that our minds & bodies don't forget: Dr. Gabor Maté - CBC Podcasts:** https://www.cbc.ca/radio/podcastnews/trauma-is-a-stupid-friend-that-our-minds-bodies-don-t-forget-dr-gabor-mat%C3%A9-1.6612920

- **Video of the letter:** https://equenergy.com/letter

- **W·I·L·D® meditations**: www.equenergy.com/meditations

- **W·I·L·D® TV YouTube channel**: https://www.youtube.com/@equenergy

- **"Four stages for learning any new skill" (Wikipedia):** https://en.wikipedia.org/wiki/Four_stages_of_competence

Examples of Power Cards I've found helpful:

» Colour cards – Secret Language of Color Cards – Inna Segal, available on Amazon
» White Lion pack – White Lion Leadership Wisdom Cards, available from https://fondation-lascaux.com/en/service/shop
» Horse pack – Available from https://equisentientcoaching.com/coaching-cards/
» Self-Love Creativity pack - By Jemma Rosenthal and BeeTee Design, from BeeTee Design on Etsy
» The Mood Cards: Make Sense of Your Moods and Emotions for Clarity, Confidence and Well-being from Andrea Harrn, available on Amazon

Books Referenced and Suggested Reading:

⇒ A H Almaas - *Diamond Heart: Elements of the Real in Man*
⇒ Bruce Lipton PhD - *The Biology of Belief*
⇒ Jack Kornfield - *The Art Of Forgiveness, Loving Kindness And Peace · 2010*
⇒ Eckart Tolle – *The Power of Now*
⇒ Neale Donald Walsch – *Conversations with God*
⇒ Dr Gabor Maté:
  * *The Myth of Normal: Trauma, Illness and Healing in a Toxic Culture*
  * *When the Body Says No*
  * *In the Realm of Hungry Ghosts*
  * *Scattered Minds: The Origins and Healing of Attention Deficit Disorder*
⇒ Bessel van der Kolk – *The Body Keeps the Score*
⇒ Andrew Cohen – *Evolutionary Enlightenment*

Books Referenced and Suggested Reading (cont):

- ⇨ J M Barrie - *Peter Pan*
- ⇨ Richard Flook - *Why Am I Sick*
- ⇨ Bronnie Ware - *The Top Five Regrets of the Dying: A Life Transformed by the Dearly Departing*
- ⇨ Clarissa Pinkola Estes – *Women Who Run With The Wolves*
- ⇨ Brené Brown:
  - * *Braving the Wilderness*
  - * *I thought it was just me*
  - * *The Gifts of Imperfection*
- ⇨ Abraham-Hicks – *The Vortex*
- ⇨ Rhonda Byrne – *The Secret*
- ⇨ Zachariah Albert - *The Law of Attraction*
- ⇨ Gemma Margerison - *Connected: The 12 Ways of Wellbeing for a Holistically Healthy Life*
- ⇨ Danny Carroll - *Terminal Cancer is a Misdiagnosis*
- ⇨ The Divine Collective - *Words of the Wise: Wisdom from Awakening Journeys*
- ⇨ Matthew Walker – *Why We Sleep*
- ⇨ *Words of the Wise - https://equenergy.com/*
- ⇨ *https://www.equenergy.com/recommended_reading/*
- ⇨ *Connected: The 12 Ways of Wellbeing for a Holistically Healthy Life - https://equenergy.com/Connected*

Useful Websites:

- ★ Robyn Harris W·I·L·D® Wellbeing: *https://www.equenergy.com*
- ★ Penny Croal, Change Ahead: *https://www.changeahead.biz*
- ★ Meta Consciousness®: *http://imca.info/*

www.ingramcontent.com/pod-product-compliance
Lightning Source LLC
Chambersburg PA
CBHW051244020426
42333CB00025B/3038